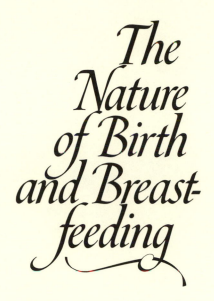

The
Nature
of Birth
and Breast-
feeding

MICHEL ODENT
The Nature of Birth and Breast-feeding

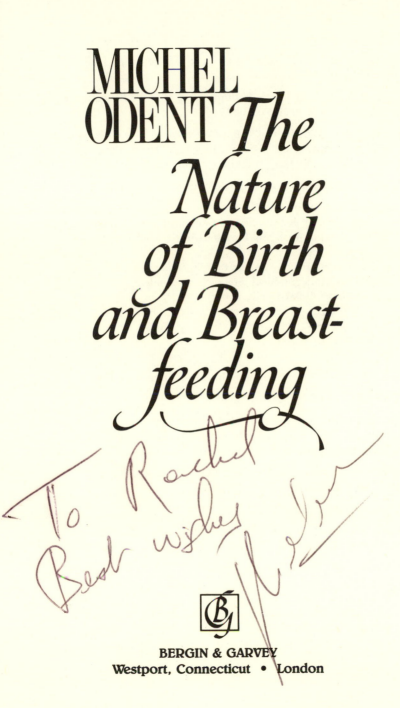

*To Rachel
Best wishes* [signature]

BERGIN & GARVEY
Westport, Connecticut • London

Copyright Acknowledgments

The author and publisher are grateful to the following for permission to quote from their material:

Priya, Jacky Vincent. *Birth Traditions and Modern Pregnancy Care.* Dorset, UK: Element Books, 1992.

Excerpt from "Midwife Cat" from *Collected and New Poems* by Mark Van Doren. Copyright © 1963 by Mark Van Doren. Reprinted by permission of Hill and Wang, a division of Farrar, Straus & Giroux, Inc.

Library of Congress Cataloging-in-Publication Data

Odent, Michel, 1930–
    [Votre bébé est le plus beau des mammifères. English]
    The nature of birth and breastfeeding / Michel Odent.
        p.   cm.
    Translation of: Votre bébé est le plus beau des mammifères.
    Includes bibliographical references and index.
    ISBN 0-89789-287-9 (alk. paper)
    1. Childbirth — Social aspects.   2. Breast feeding — Social aspects.
I. Title.
RG652.03413   1992
304.6'3 — dc20   91-44076

British Library Cataloguing in Publication Data is available.

Library of Congress Catalog Card Number: 91-44076
ISBN: 0-89789-287-9

First published in 1992

Bergin & Garvey, 88 Post Road West, Westport, CT 06881
An imprint of Greenwood Publishing Group, Inc.

Printed in the United States of America

∞™

The paper used in this book complies with the Permanent Paper Standard issued by the National Information Standards Organization (Z39.48-1984).

10 9 8 7 6 5 4 3

Contents

Acknowledgments

I owe thanks:

to the countless mothers, babies, and other anonymous contributors to this book.

to Alice Charlwood, my linguistic adviser.

to Sophy Craze. Her precious advice is inspired by her experience as an editor, as a writer, and as a mother.

to Nancy Cohen. The *"Open Season"* was hardly over when she agreed to read my manuscript and wrote pages of authoritative comments full of "Nancyisms."

Introduction to the American Edition

Attitudes toward childbirth in the 1990s abound in paradoxes:

- On the one hand, it has been widely demonstrated that the only effect of electronic fetal monitoring on childbirth statistics is to increase the rate of cesarean sections. On the other hand, most babies in the industrialized countries are born in an electronic environment.
- On the one hand, some of the most impressive childbirth statistics, with low rates of cesarean section, come out of Holland — the only developed country where as many as one baby in every three is born at home. On the other hand, pregnant women all over the world are commonly told that home birth is dangerous.
- On the one hand, births in Western countries where midwives are numerous and well established have the best outcomes, with low rates of cesarean section. On the other hand, it is in precisely those countries where the number of cesareans has reached epidemic proportions that midwifery is most devalued or even threatened with extinction.
- On the one hand, many administrators and public

health specialists are desperately in search of strategies to reduce the cost of medical treatment. On the other hand, it has been calculated that the cost of electronic fetal monitoring in the United States is about $400 million per year.

• On the one hand, there is now serious concern about the suspected long-term ill effects of the drugs used during labor, especially with regard to cancer and drug addiction. On the other hand, there is no general tendency to reduce the use of these drugs.

The existence of so many paradoxes is typical of a period of transition. By becoming more scientific, obstetrics is discovering its own limitations and is finally evaluating the power of the environment in the period surrounding birth.

The ecology of breastfeeding is also becoming topical at a time when scientists are more and more convinced of the irreplaceable value of human milk. The main concern among public health agencies is the current short duration of breastfeeding. Why do only a tiny minority of mothers still breastfeed when the baby is six months old, although the majority of them breastfeed at birth? Some health authorities are aware of the importance of the attitude of society as a whole. These authorities could do much to influence the duration of breastfeeding by encouraging policies that would allow longer parental leaves of absence from work, for instance, as they do in Sweden. They could also try to make more facilities available for mothers who will be breastfeeding in public places such as shops and highway service stations. This is the meaning of the recommendations published by the British Minister of Health.

But it is commonplace to tackle this issue without putting it into the context of our very special society, characterized by the small, monogamous, nuclear family. The duration of breastfeeding and the family structure are two topics we should never dissociate. Therefore, in due time, we will dare in this book to raise the basic question that is all too often evaded: Is prolonged breastfeeding compatible (at a cultural level) with the monogamous, nuclear family?

In the field of childbirth and breastfeeding, we should constantly refer to our mammalian roots and our mammalian needs. That is why this book was originally written for the French. For many of them, it is still a challenging idea to think of humans as mammals. For English-speaking people, the same idea is not nearly so provocative. If you tell them that they are mammals, most of them do not mind. They do not even react — as if you were stating the obvious. But then look at the childbirthing facts to the contrary. Look at the way babies are born and fed in English-speaking countries. Their basic needs are no better met there than in France. In some conventional hospitals, it is difficult to imagine how the mammalian need for privacy might be even taken into consideration. It is routine to delay the first skin-to-skin contact between mother and baby, and the beginning of breastfeeding is disturbed in many ways. Even the advocates of so-called natural childbirth focus on the needs for support, for help, for assistance. The universal need for privacy is not stressed; or if it is mentioned, it is not really understood.

More generally speaking, a majority of cultures the world over have found excuses to deny the need for privacy in the period of time surrounding birth. One of their most universal justifications for this is to claim that colostrum is bad for the baby. This belief probably had an evolutionary advantage in the past as an effective way of distorting the relationship between mother and newborn. Cross-cultural comparisons suggest a link between the quality of the mother-baby relationship and respect for Mother Earth. They also suggest that the capacity to dominate any and all forms of life has been more important for the survival of many human groups than their respect for Mother Earth.

Now the priorities are different. Weakening respect for the planet and interfering in the mother-baby relationship cannot be advantageous any more. To recognize the need for privacy and rediscover the truly natural childbirth, we have to go beyond obstetrics and the current practices of midwifery.

This is the reason why I found it relevant to publish a translation of the original French text.

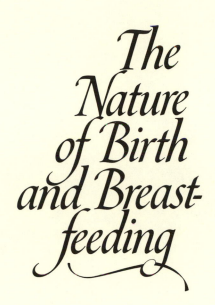

The
Nature
of Birth
and Breast-
feeding

CHAPTER ONE

Our Mammalian Roots

I have received, Sir, your new book against the human race. . . . Nobody has ever used more intelligence in an attempt to turn us into beasts; reading your book gives one the desire to walk on all fours!
—Letter from Voltaire to Rousseau after reading
"Discours sur l'inégalité," 1755

One hundred years before Darwin, Jean Jacques Rousseau dared to include human beings in the animal kingdom. Voltaire and the French intellectuals concealed behind irony their incapacity to understand his ideas.

More than a hundred years after Darwin, Voltaire lives on. I meet him during any of my visits to France. I have lived outside France almost permanently since 1985, so now I am only a visitor. The experience of home birth I have acquired in England has been both fruitful and necessary. How can you understand the effects of the environment on the process of birth and the first contact between mother and baby if you do not change your own surroundings, cultural and linguistic? I had to progress beyond what I had learned in the context of a French hospital, so as to become aware of the actual potential of a woman in labor, and to distinguish what is fundamental, universal, from what is contingent and linked with local custom.

This is how I often summarize my twenty-five years of research: "I learned that human beings are mammals. All mammals hide themselves, isolate themselves to give birth. They need privacy. It is the same for humans. We should always be aware of this need for privacy."

This point of view is easily accepted in the English-speaking countries. It is considered merely common sense. But if you express the same idea in France, even in the most cautious terms, you immediately get a dismayed response in a distinctly Voltairian tone: "But we are not animals." "We are not rats." "We are human beings empowered by language." "Our capacity for symbolism . . ." "Our integration in a cultural milieu . . ." "Our awareness of our own mortality . . ." And so on.

"Humans are mammals" — a cliché!

Les êtres humains sont des mammifères" — a provocative statement!

It is common among many French intellectuals to see the human phenomenon as that which makes us different from the rest of the animal kingdom, and to ignore the depth of our roots. However, a clear awareness of what we are would not be repressed, or delayed, if we could overcome this arrogance. Let us reflect anew on the eloquent lesson in humility we could learn from the one who decided to be born in a stable 2,000 years ago.

The main proposition of ecological science is that all forms of life are interdependent; and, even as ecological awareness is becoming the most important event of this century, we have to be wary of our old Voltairian reflexes.

"Voltaire: the end of a world. Rousseau: the beginning of a new one." Goethe's prophecy takes on a whole new meaning if we consider it in the context of the birth of human beings, in which case the rediscovery of our animal roots seems even more urgent and necessary. Mammals are characterized by the way they are born and fed as infants. The story began some 200 million years ago when a little animal developed in the belly of its mother before entering the world.

To give birth to their offspring through the process of delivery, female mammals have to secrete a number of hormones. These same hormones are at work in the delivery of human babies. They are secreted by the brain's most primitive structures — those that we share with all mammals. These similarities should be the starting point whenever we try to improve our understanding of the process of birth in our species.

That is, we *need* to start from this point; but by and large, we don't. Enormous credibility has been given to attitudes about birth that support basic misunderstandings regarding the physiological processes. The French are responsible for the most significant errors. Fernand Lamaze, the father of the so-called Lamaze method, used to say that a woman has to learn to give birth in the same way that we learn to speak, or to read, or to swim. This erroneous thinking has been accepted everywhere in the world and, finally, has led to our current crisis.

The words of the American obstetrician Robert Austin Bradley are significantly similar to those of Lamaze, and serve as an example of the deadlock in which we find ourselves. He compared the situation of a pregnant woman with a woman who is given nine months' notice that she will be thrown into deep water. Of course, this woman would use the nine months in learning how to swim. In the same way, a pregnant woman should learn how to give birth.

When you consider birth as an involuntary process involving old, primitive, mammalian structures of the brain, you set aside the assumption that a woman must learn how to give birth. It is implicit in the mammalian interpretation that one cannot actively help a woman to give birth. The goal is to avoid disturbing her unnecessarily.

All over the world, there are women who are trying to counterbalance the dominant intellectual attitude. In the English-speaking countries, the most concrete form of reaction has been in the work of many new-style childbirth educators. For the most part, these are mothers who have no special qualification but, having given birth to their own children, feel the need to help other women who could benefit from their personal experience. They organize meetings, often at their own homes. They do not usually encumber themselves with any particular theoretical basis for their teaching, but may find it useful to give this or that school of thought as a reference. Their aim could most accurately be described as being to provide information and education, rather than specific preparation.

In a society characterized by the small nuclear family and birth in hospitals, these new childbirth educators endeavor to satisfy the social needs of pregnant women: their need to meet other pregnant women, mothers, and babies. They play the educational role that was traditionally played by the mother, aunts, and other women of the older generations. They fill a gap peculiar to our society, which tends to separate one generation of mothers from the next.

In the United States, I met some of these promoters of a different kind of birth. They play an important educational role without calling themselves "educators." The story of one of them deserves to be told.

When she was a little girl living on her parents' farm in North Dakota, her father gave her the responsibility of being present when the baby pigs were born. And he told her what to do: "Don't show yourself. Stay hidden. If the sow feels watched the delivery will be longer, more difficult, more dangerous; and after the birth, she might have no interest in her babies. She might even become aggressive. So make yourself inconspicuous — but be aware of what is happening. Although the sow is the most competent mother imaginable, she might accidentally neglect or suffocate one of her eight or ten or more babies. If this happens, you should intervene discreetly and tactfully, only to protect the safety of the little pigs by moving them out of harm's way and returning them to suckle once the sow has again lain down on her side."

When this little girl grew up, she had children of her own. To give birth, she went to a hospital for humans and had to lie down on a table, surrounded by experts who were telling her to push, or not to push, or to breathe in this way or that. She discovered that they knew nothing about birth, and she became conscious of the considerable merit in the advice given to her by her father. So she started to organize seminars, workshops, and conferences to change the way babies are born. And that is why I visited North Dakota.

She is typical of a growing number of women who — independently of professional experts — have accumulated a huge potential for criticism and creativity over the years that is still latent and untapped. The countries where rates of cesareans have reached absurd proportions and where obstetricians are obsessed with malpractice suits are also, paradoxically, the best suited to generate radical change.

In France, such childbirth educators are unknown. Formally qualified experts monopolize the so-called preparation for childbirth and are reimbursed by the state system of social welfare. The lack of vocational childbirth educators and the intellectual attitude that focuses on the divide between humans and the animal kingdom are two expressions of an incapacity to raise simple questions. When I am outside my own country, I find it easier to understand the difficulties that are specifically French.

At the beginning of the 1980s, my priority had been to write a book for the American public. Today I am writing for the French public first. But why today?

CHAPTER TWO

At the Dawn of the Post-Electronic Age

During the past two decades, most Western babies were born in an electronic environment. Obstetricians had arrived at the theory that if they could record the rhythm of the baby's heartbeat continuously during labor with electronic machines they would be in an ideal situation to rescue some babies in danger, should the need arise. They were convinced that this would be the way to make births safer. In fact, however, it was only a belief, not supported by scientific evidence.

Many recent events suggest that the electronic age of birthing might be drawing to a close. We are at a turning point in the history of childbirth. A turning point means a change of direction that can be pinpointed quite precisely. I believe the relevant date in this case was December 12, 1987, when an important article was published in *Lancet*, one of the most authoritative medical journals in the world. This article compared eight studies conducted in Australia, the United States, and Europe that had involved tens of thousands of births and had compared groups of women giving birth with electronic fetal monitoring with other groups of women giving birth with a midwife who merely listened intermittently to the baby's heartbeat. Several of these studies had been published previously in the most prestigious medical journals, such as the *New England Journal of Medicine;* but the *Lancet* article brought all the various documents together for the first time. The overall conclusion reached was that the only statistically significant effect of electronic fetal-heart monitoring is to increase the rate of cesareans and forceps deliveries. No significant difference could be shown between the two groups when comparing the number of babies alive at birth and the number of babies healthy at birth. The only possible interpretation of these findings must be that the use of electronic monitoring during labor is dangerous. It makes the birth more difficult. More babies need to be rescued by more operations. Thanks to the data vouchsafed by the most serious and orthodox medical literature, these facts are known everywhere in the world.[1] We now need to be fully aware of all its implications.

This means that the declining infant mortality rates for the period around birth (which became evident around the beginning of this century and continued during the past three decades) must be explained by reasons other than the routine use of continuous electronic monitoring. There is now no excuse for requiring all babies to be born in an electronic environment. More generally speaking, the time has come to consider the effects of the environment on the process of birth and the first contact between mother and baby. We must start raising new and simple questions and preparing ourselves for the post-electronic age.

For many doctors these findings are difficult to integrate with their beliefs and their style of practice. But for some midwives and women, and even for some doctors, the findings reported in *Lancet* (and elsewhere) merely confirm what is obvious. At the beginning of the 1970s I requested the purchase of an electronic fetal-heart monitoring machine in our hospital, thinking that, in some cases, the additional information it provided would help us to avoid unnecessary cesareans. After a three-month trial period, Dominique — the most experienced midwife on our team — returned her verdict: "This is just a device to increase the number of cesareans." If the need for privacy, and the need not to feel observed and controlled had been better understood, the effects of continuous monitoring might have been foreseen and the electronic illusion avoided.

People who are studying in a medical school, or a conventional European midwifery school, are trained to answer certain questions. They are also trained to avoid certain other questions. But it is urgent to ask and answer these other questions now. What kind of environment can inhibit a woman in labor? What kind of environment can disturb the first contact between mother and baby, and the beginning of breastfeeding?

These are simple and new key questions that we are obliged to address during this period of transition. Let us translate them into medical jargon, or even into a topic for an examination question: "What kinds of environmental factors inhibit human parturition?" Medical students have never had to reflect on this question in an exam. How would they be able to collect the appropriate data? The textbooks would not be of any help — at least the textbooks about humans. But medical students might take their inspiration from information gathered by scientists who have been studying the birth of other mammals; these scientists formulated the question exactly as we have, and found some interesting answers.

The most significant studies were those carried out by Niles Newton in Chicago, who spent part of her career in the 1960s evaluating the effects of the environment on the birth of nonhuman mammals. She studied the birth of mice in particular and tried to analyze the environmental factors that make their deliveries longer, more difficult, and more dangerous. Through her work we can learn the most efficient strategies to make birth more difficult. One might, for instance, place the laboring female in an unfamiliar environment — a place where the sights and smells are not what she is used to in her daily life. Or one might move the mother-to-be from one place to another during labor. Another experiment demonstrated that a transparent cage made of glass also tends to increase the difficulties. This scientific approach suggests that mammals prefer to hide themselves when giving birth to their offspring. They need privacy.

After studying the effects of environment on the birth of human babies for several decades, I am convinced that all Niles Newton's findings also apply to our species. Fortunately, I became aware of the importance of her work early enough to be able to understand a variety of human behaviors during the period surrounding birth. I have also borrowed some of her favorite phrases, such as "fetus ejection reflex." When I compare the works of scientists like her with what I have learned about the birth of humans, all my doubts vanish. We are mammals. We have to make up for the time lost through our obsession about differences between species. We should not feel ashamed to admit that other mammals can help us to rediscover what some of us have forgotten. And one thing that human cultures in the West have forgotten, or want to forget, is the need for privacy of the woman giving birth and welcoming her baby.

It is not absolutely necessary to refer to the scientific experiments to be aware of mammals' need for privacy. In fact, this is a much observed and well-known feature of mammalian behavior, both in those whose young are already relatively mature and autonomous at birth like the bovines and sheep, and those who are not mature at all, like the rats. For example the pregnant sheep, normally a herd dweller, separates herself from the flock when birth becomes imminent. A female bighorn sheep will seek out the most inaccessible spot on the mountain and may stay there, isolated, for days without food and water while awaiting her newborn. The rhesus monkey moves away from her group to the edge of the forest and picks a well-camouflaged hiding place so that she may give birth alone, away from the curious eyes and unwanted attentions of other group members.

Even mammals that do not have the option of moving away from the group still try to isolate themselves. The rat — normally a nocturnal prowler — gives birth during the day; and the horse — normally a daytime grazer — gives birth during the night.

Why do mammals hide themselves, isolate themselves, to give birth? Why this universal need for privacy? Obviously, the aim is not to protect themselves against predators. If this were the priority, regrouping would occur. The females hide themselves to be protected against the other members of their own group. And why? That question is the reason for this book, and is too important to be answered right away.

Let us return first to some practical considerations that are unique to our time. Is it possible to maintain an atmosphere of privacy in a maternity hospital? How might it be possible? These are basic questions for the advent of the post-electronic age.

Note

1. Similar results have been obtained from studies that focus on specific aspects of the birth experience, such as electronic fetal monitoring before the labor starts, or electronic fetal monitoring during premature deliveries. See the Selected Bibliography for a list of the articles that suggest the electronic age in birthing is drawing to a close.

CHAPTER THREE

The Hospital of the Future

The birthing centers or maternity hospitals of the future will probably have very little in common with the obstetric departments of the electronic age. Of course, they will be attached to a hospital — in close proximity to a building where a medical team will be at the service of women and midwives, day and night, and ready to perform that wonderful operation called the cesarean section, if it should suddenly become necessary.

A cesarean section, performed with the current surgical techniques and the assistance of modern anesthesia, represents the main advance in the field of childbirth this century. This is the kind of advance worth preserving. It is a model, a reference for any other rescue operation. Any emergency surgical team should be able to do it, but it should not become the usual way to be born. It should not become an excuse for maintaining our ignorance of the physiological processes of birth.

How can we provide an atmosphere of privacy in a birthing center or maternity hospital? Is it possible for mothers not to feel observed and controlled in such places? How can this be done?

Everyone knows that it is easier to have a feeling of privacy in a familiar place; this is common knowledge, even among those who do not know about our mammalian nature and have not heard about experiments with mice! The prime aim should be to enable the mother-to-be to gain familiarity with the birthing place. She must be helped to feel at home. It is not enough to have had a guided tour of the facilities and to be told the whereabouts of the midwives' desk, the birthing room, or the TV room. In order to become really familiar with a place you have to be there often and keep coming there to do something. And it is better still if you are doing something pleasant. In the future, all birth attendants who are concerned with giving priority to the need for privacy must think about the sorts of activities adapted to pregnant women that could be developed in a birthing center. The important thing is to ask the questions. A variety of answers will be found according to the time, the premises, the kind of population being served, as well as the personality of the people in charge of the center.

We found an answer that was perfectly adapted to our maternity hospital in Pithiviers, France. The pregnant women and the staff would meet and sing around the piano! What could be easier, or more pleasant? It wasn't expensive. Somebody calculated that you can buy twelve secondhand pianos for the price of an electronic fetal monitor.

I could talk at length about those singing sessions. Singing can be looked on as a breathing exercise. In another context it can be considered as a fundamental human need — a cross-cultural need that becomes difficult to meet in our age of professional singers, of the media and the sophistication of recording techniques. Again, singing can be looked at from the point of view of the fetus whose vibratory sense is precociously mature and needs stimulation. Bearing in mind the popularity of singing in groups, let us remember that humans are social animals and that the social needs of pregnant women and young mothers are satisfied at all the wrong times in our society. Pregnant women and breastfeeding mothers are usually isolated at a time when they need strong social support; and women in labor are surrounded by three or four people at a time when they most need privacy.

So let us go back to the need for privacy. When we are in a place where we have shared not only ideas but also emotions, either by singing or dancing, we become attached to the place itself. The place, as well as the people, become familiar. In retrospect I find it difficult to imagine any activities better suited to changing the mental pictures we usually associate with the word *hospital*. Provided that all the members of the team — the midwives, nurses, doctors, and secretaries — mingle with parents, babies, children, and even grandparents, this approach always works.

Many details easily linked with the idea of privacy are important when giving birth. When a laboring woman arrives at the birthing center or maternity hospital she should, ideally, immediately occupy the room that will be her territory in the hours up to and immediately following the birth. Just as Niles Newton's mice had a longer, more difficult, and more dangerous labor when they were moved from one place to another, all midwives know that having to move a mother from a labor room to a separate delivery room often results in the delivery's being postponed. Modern women giving birth in any kind of birthing center or hospital spend some time in at least three different places: first at home when the labor starts; then in a car; and then, finally, in the building where the baby will be born.

In the United States, I have visited one maternity hospital where the birthing rooms had a lot in common with ours in Pithiviers, but — even better — there were enough of these rooms so that each woman could go immediately to one of them and stay there until the birth and even afterward. Our *salle sauvage* in Pithiviers has often been depicted and imitated. In the mid-1970s it was absolutely new to design, in a state hospital, a birthing room where the dominant colors were brown or cream — and unheard of that the room should have no medical equipment, and no bed or table that would impose one particular labor position. There are some details about our homelike birthing place that I should have stressed more insistently in the past, but it was only when I had had experience of home birth that I understood their actual importance. It seems paradoxical to claim that only those with experience of home birth can design the hospitals of the future. In any case, I only became really aware of the importance of the size of the birthing room quite recently.

Once more, one must refer to the behavior of other mammals, who usually try to find a small corner or a small intimate space where it is easier to feel private. At home it is tempting to prepare the place of birth and locate it in advance, if only to protect the carpets! But, quite often, the baby is born somewhere nobody had foreseen, and it is always in the smallest possible room — for example, a child's bedroom, or the bathroom. I have always wondered why taking a shower can seem more efficient than taking a bath; just perhaps, it is because the shower is usually tucked away in a tiny corner. A woman once told me, "My dream is to give birth in a cupboard." Another couple had protected in advance the beautiful carpet covering the floor of their huge bedroom. At the last minute the mother-to-be rushed into a corner behind the piano, hung from a coat hook, and dropped her nine-pound baby on the only spot where the carpet was unprotected! In Italy I visited a birthing room that was an enlarged copy of the one in Pithiviers, but the atmosphere was totally different — much more awe inspiring and intimidating.

Is giving birth easier in a small room or a large one? This is the sort of new, simple, and fruitful question that immediately comes up when humans are classified among the mammals. There is another detail that I now find much more important than I could have imagined in the past: there is a point at which a certain amount of disorder can reinforce an atmosphere of privacy. After visiting an obstetric unit, a midwife and I were trying to analyze why we had not felt at ease in the place. The reason was simple: everything was in perfect order. Few people noticed in Pithiviers that I used to make a discreet round of the facilities every day just to create a bit of disorder. At the time I was just following an unconscious intuition, but today I dare to talk about it openly. When I am called to a home birth and immediately feel at home, I now know why.

A small room, a small corner, a few things out of place — let us add another detail that would be completely unthinkable if your point of reference is a delivery room of the electronic age. Yet again, we are simply rediscovering what most mammals know instinctively: one does not feel so observed in the dark. Most female mammals try to find a dim corner to give birth to their offspring, and darkness may be even more important for the birth of humans than for many other mammals. Nevertheless, even some home birth midwives who are very careful to disturb the birth as little as possible have a tendency to underestimate the importance of a dimmed light.

The birth process is a brain process. In labor and delivery, the primitive part of the brain that we share with all other mammals is active. This part of the brain must secrete the hormones necessary for efficient uterine contractions, but its functions can be inhibited just as they can be during all the other events of the sexual life. These inhibitions come from the new brain, the neocortex, which enables us to be rational, scientific, and to communicate through language. The release of the hormones necessary for the birth process is accompanied by a reduction in the activity of the new brain; and that is why, at a certain stage of a normal physiological birth, women seem to divorce themselves from their surroundings and attendants and drift off to another planet. Their level of consciousness changes, as it must if they are to reach the right hormonal balance. On the other hand, you can stop the progress of labor by stimulating the neocortex and asking the mother-to-be something like "What is your Social Security number?"

Light, too, is a well-known stimulus to the neocortex. This is well understood by those who explore the electric activity of the brain by electroencephalography. The sense of sight is the most intellectual of our senses. From this, one can deduce the special importance of darkness during human labor. Since human beings are characterized by the huge development of their neocortex — the part of the brain that inhibits the instinctive, involuntary processes — we can begin to understand that darkness is probably even more important for the birth of humans than it is for the birth of other mammals. It is precisely this development of the neocortex that makes all instinctive human behavior so fragile, so dependent on the environment. Of course, many people don't need a long explanation to convince them that closing the curtains tends to reinforce the feeling of privacy.

Making the place familiar, taking the size of the birthing room into account, being aware of the advantages of a certain amount of disorder and of darkness — it is easy to satisfy all these requirements. One just has to be aware of their importance. And any maternity hospital could be adapted to accommodate them overnight.

Of course, nurturing a long-term vision will bring up other questions. What suggestions should be made to the architects commissioned to design the maternity centers of the future? What sort of size should they be? Should there be a few huge centers welcoming thousands of babies a year, or very many small centers handling only a few hundred births a year? Will the current angular shapes of the buildings give way to more rounded lines? In this age of concrete, even birthing places are made of materials synthesized by man.

Perhaps organic materials such as clay, wood, or simply brick will be preferred — breathing materials, capable of transmitting humidity from inside to outside and vice versa. Perhaps people will be concerned about the electromagnetic environment, looking at the location of the center in relation to a nearby electrified railway or high-voltage cables as well as considering the building materials and the geophysical situation.

The new generation of architects tends now to consider the interaction of a building with both its environment and the people who work or live within it. Some modern buildings might be damaging to the personal health of their occupants, and we learn that this curse — the so-called sick building syndrome — might result from the rapid development of building material technology.

The important thing, as always, is to be asking the questions. The answers will follow.

CHAPTER FOUR

On Another Planet

And what about the human environment in the birthing centers of the future? Since the word *privacy* means the state of not being observed, or not feeling observed, the presence of people during the birth is at the very heart of the matter.

Most mammals have settled the question in the simplest possible way: they hide themselves; they isolate themselves.

It is likely that many humans living in cultures remote from ours have had the same attitude. In a film made by Wulf Schiefenhovel of a birth among the Eipos, a tribe of New Guinea, we see how the mothers-to-be go to the bush when they are about to give birth. Isolating oneself in this way has been the rule in societies as far afield as the Turkomans in Central Asia and tribes of Canadian Indians, for example. It is notable that, in those very societies where women tend to isolate themselves to give birth, the deliveries are reputed to be easy.

But this is not the case in most human societies that have survived up to the present day. In most of these cultures — including ours until quite recently — women have always tried to protect themselves from at least the presence of men. Giving birth was women's business. Of course, men have always tried to accord themselves some importance in the period surrounding birth. Thus, most societies have, at a certain stage of their evolution, come to the same compromise in this struggle — channeling the emotional reactions of the father, satisfying his need to play a role, and, at the same time, keeping him outside. This is what is commonly called the *couvade*, meaning that the husband imitates his wife in labor. In some places he is responsible for presenting the baby to the community; he can be looked after or receive congratulations. Women have also long tolerated the intrusion of men on the occasion of such ceremonies as circumcision or baptism. However, from the seventeenth century on, it became more and more common for a male doctor to intrude into the birthing room.

The newest phenomenon in this compromising of birth's privacy — a phenomenon that started in the middle of this century — was almost unheard of in the prior history of humanity and even in the history of the mammals. Suddenly, many women felt a need for the participation of the father at the birth of their baby. This was really new. At the beginning of this century, before hospital birth became so commonplace, the baby's father was only present somewhere in the house and kept busy with practical tasks, such as filling huge basins of water.

At that time the attitude of the man could not really have been called "participation." Childbirth was still firmly the woman's domain. But what is happening now can only be interpreted by recalling how it started. The participation of the baby's father began when more and more births started taking place in the hospital. At around the same time, the role of the midwife underwent a crucial change: she either became an anonymous member of the medical team or disappeared altogether. As these things were happening, the size of the family was also being reduced to the dimensions of today's nuclear family.

We are still too close to have a proper view of these phenomena, but they do provoke new concerns. The issue of
the human environment during a birth is more complicated
than ever, but some simple rules can be easily summarized.
Aphoristically, we might say, "The length of labor is propor-
tional to the number of people around."

To take stock of the complexity of this issue and the
countless variety of situations that can occur, let us consider
some scenarios that I have come across, both at home and in
the hospital. The point I want to emphasize is that, with
sufficient experience, it is often possible to guess at once
whether a birth is likely to be long and difficult or fast and
easy, just with a glance or a brief peep through a crack in
the door. I learn a lot from my first impression when I enter
a house for a home birth. For example, if the woman has
locked herself in her bathroom, it is a good sign. The baby
will probably be born soon. Unfortunately, this highly significant behavior tends to make members of the hospital
team very jumpy. They would find it necessary to knock on
the door and shout, "Don't do that!" And, "What if the
baby comes and you cannot open the door?"

And when I see a laboring woman on the floor — about to
go off to another planet — and nobody around except a midwife reading a newspaper, I am also optimistic. An experienced midwife does not need to disturb the mother's
privacy in labor by repeated vaginal exams. She does not
need to behave like an observer. By "experienced midwife" I
mean a midwife who is familiar with women whose labor
need not be "managed," who feel free to be noisy, to breathe
the way they want to, and to adopt any position. Just by listening, the midwife will know more about how the labor is
progressing than she could by probing with her finger.

When the mother-to-be is alone with the baby's father
and he seems to really share the emotions, leaving our world
at the same time as his wife — a scene that would have been
considered unbelievable fifty years ago — it is also possible

that the birth will not be too long away or too difficult. In this case, once more, nobody behaves like an observer. It is not the woman who is giving birth; it is the couple.

The issue is very different when the man places himself in front of his wife and tends to look her in the eye. It is as if, when his wife is ready to shift into another level of consciousness, he were saying, "Stay with me." Eye-to-eye contact is a powerful means of communication between human beings. There are occasions when the aim is specifically to take advantage of this power — as, for example, when a therapist encourages an autistic child to meet the eyes of his or her mother during a so-called holding session. But when a woman is in labor, this is counterproductive. When a man places himself in front of his wife, he behaves like an observer and also puts himself in a position of control, ready to suggest this or that position or this or that way to breathe. When that happens, you can anticipate a long and difficult birth. The situation is, of course, worsened when several people are around behaving like observers — and maybe someone there waving a camera!

Some women are able to hide from the whole world so that the behavior of their partner and other attendants does not matter, whatever the context. I know a woman who had a fast first delivery in a busy hospital after hiding under a towel. For the birth of her second baby she was at home, hiding under a dressing gown.

If the behavior of the attendants does not really matter in such circumstances, their mere presence can nevertheless be important. There is no privacy without a feeling of security. Privacy has to be protected.

I have a special interest in the attitude of some men who tend to stay close to the birthing room, seeming to protect the privacy of their wife from outside. If somebody wants to enter the room, it is as if they were saying with a wave of the hand or with one or two words, "No, not now. She is giving birth."

In spite of all the current social pressures suggesting that the man must participate in the birth, these young men seem to have rediscovered one of the original male roles: to protect the women and babies against other human groups and all sorts of predators.

At a time when there is a lot of stress on immediate father-baby bonding — by encouraging the father to communicate with the baby even in the womb, and to share the experience of birth, and all in the framework of the small nuclear family — it might be fruitful to look a little more closely at the role of the man as protector, and once more to refer to our condition as primates.

In the world of primates, the attachment between father and baby seems usually to develop via the mother. The male tends to protect the females he has mated with, and their babies. His lack of aggression toward the baby, if not attachment, is derived from the mother's interest. It is perhaps more dangerous than we commonly believe to copy too closely the father-infant bonding from the mother-infant bonding, when the hormonal basis of these two processes is so different. Father-infant bonding needs time and is built up gradually. It follows a chronological pattern that we will probably have to relearn and take into account.

I remember hundreds of wonderful births in which the father was deeply involved. This obviously reinforced the comradeship between the couple, but perhaps not the sexual interest. Still, it was sometimes followed a year or so later by an amicable divorce, and the child subsequently shared by both parents on equal terms.

It is most important to acknowledge the complexity of this topic and to avoid the temptation to create a lot of new rules. I know women who did not dare to admit that, at a certain stage of labor, they would have preferred their husbands to take a walk around the park. And, of course, there have also been men who felt obliged to participate in the birth simply out of obedience to the current social trend.

Many modern women insist that they would not have been able to give birth without the support of their husbands, and many men consider the birth of the baby to have been their most enriching and rewarding experience. In fact, therefore, each is a particular case: there are couples who are still in the phase of seduction, couples threatened by a hidden conflict, couples who have intimately shared their lives for fifteen years, couples where the dominant partner is the man, others where the dominant person is the woman, as well as single mothers. It will take many decades to distinguish the attitudes peculiar to the electronic age in the history of childbirth, from those modern views that will stand the test of time.

In any case, if we are to sweep away the legacy of the era that is drawing to a close, and build a new basis for birthing care, we must concentrate on this issue of the man's place — an issue whose importance has not yet been fully appreciated. Indeed, why was it that, in the past, laboring women always tried to protect themselves from the presence of men? Several interpretations could be mooted, and they do corroborate each other.

First, we could claim that it was a way of cultivating the mystery of femininity and childbirth for the men. Sexual attraction subsists on mystery. This interpretation is supported by recent inquiries such as those made by Sam Janus in New York, who found that there is a high proportion of men who are impotent after participating in the birth of their babies. Actually, this amounts to a lack of sexual interest in their own wives. However, is this really a negative effect if you consider that prolactin, the hormone of lactation, tends to reduce the sex drive of the breastfeeding mother? Perhaps, in general terms, we are raising here an issue that is peculiar to our monogamous nuclear families.

Second, we should also consider that during the past several million years human beings have had to master the most dangerous animals on Earth. Clans have eliminated other clans. Tribes have eliminated other tribes. Civilizations have dominated or eliminated other civilizations. The only human groups we can study directly or indirectly on this planet are the descendants of those who successfully maximized their aggressive potential and became the best hunters and the best warriors. Sharing the emotions of a scene of birth is not exactly compatible with the education of a man whose mission is to kill calmly, should the occasion arise. A squadron of the mobile military state police force is based in Pithiviers. Seeing some of those young men bursting into tears at the birth of their baby, we all felt how difficult it must have been to reconcile such an experience with the capacity to fulfil their particular social function.

This idea suggests that keeping men away from the scene of birth has been an advantage so long as the priority has been to dominate the other species and other human groups. But everything has to be reconsidered when the survival of the planet becomes the priority.

The interpretation of the man's-place issue that I tend to put forward (without disavowing the others) takes our mammalian nature into consideration first. It is likely that women originally isolated themselves to give birth, perhaps calling for help, with a typical scream if help was needed during the very last contractions. The need for privacy has been gradually denied throughout our history. Giving birth in the company of other women was a first stage of this evolution. Today, with the introduction of the medical man, with the masculine connotation of the word *technology,* with the trend toward imposing the participation of the baby's father and the common belief that a woman cannot give birth without a support person, we have reached the nadir in terms of acknowledging the need for privacy. However, at the same time, people are beginning to be aware of the absurdity of the situation. We have to go back to square one and remember that we are primarily mammals.

An anecdote made me conscious of the irony of the

present situation. A group of women in a small American city was talking about a local obstetrician who was thought to be more "human" than his colleagues. He understood that women need a degree of privacy when giving birth, and would stay in the background and dim the lights; he did not seek to impose any position or breathing pattern, and did not cut short the first skin-to-skin contact between mother and baby; he had a special interest in breastfeeding. "By the way," a woman added ingenuously, "he used to be a veterinarian."

In France more than anywhere else, we are strongly attracted to and influenced by the so-called human sciences: sociology, linguistics, ethnology, psychoanalysis, history. Fundamentally, their *raison d'être* is the gap between humanity and the rest of the animal kingdom. But when the birth of our babies is concerned, when one is aware of the common roots in many languages of the word *nature* and the word meaning to be born (e.g., *naître*), it is first and foremost toward the science of the mammals that one should turn.

CHAPTER FIVE

The Fetus Ejection Reflex

Love-making begins with caresses and ends like a fight.
F. Leboyer

As soon as one becomes aware of the importance of the word *privacy* and its real meaning, it is necessary to observe some simple rules that command our attention. These principles remain the same at every stage of labor: the first stage, during which the cervix gradually dilates; the second stage, which culminates in the delivery of the baby; and the third stage, which is the period from the delivery of the infant to the recovery of the placenta. But, in an atmosphere of complete privacy, of perfect spontaneity, when the mother-to-be is in a small dark room and does not feel observed, these different stages have few points in common with the features that have been described in the textbooks for midwives and doctors over the past three centuries. Most obstetricians cannot begin to imagine what a birth might be like when it is not controlled and observed. The most characteristic phase of a delivery in "the method of the mammals" is around the time of the very last contractions before the baby is born, when what I call "the fetus ejection reflex" is manifest.

Until recently the term *fetus ejection reflex* had been used only by the American scientist Niles Newton with reference to nonhuman mammals. But she had imagined as early as the 1960s that one day the phrase might become as relevant to a good understanding of the process of human parturition as the phrase *milk ejection reflex* (or *let-down reflex*) is for a good understanding of lactation. I am now convinced that Niles Newton was right. If one day the art of midwifery is truly rediscovered, it will be inseparable from the practice of not hindering the fetus ejection reflex.

Many people do not like this phrase at first. My main reason for finding it perfectly appropriate is that it facilitates a parallel with the "milk ejection reflex" and the "sperm ejection reflex." Newton's vocabulary itself helps us to understand that the different episodes of the sexual life tend to follow roughly the same patterns. Also, Niles Newton is a mother who has a deep understanding of childbirth and breastfeeding. One cannot fairly claim that her terminology is masculine. It is scientific.

The word *reflex* first recommended itself to me in very special circumstances. We had observed that immersion in a pool full of warm water was an effective way of facilitating the phase of dilation of the cervix. So long as the mother-to-be does not get into the bath until the onset of hard contractions in the middle of this phase, we learnt to expect that once immersed she would be fully dilated quite quickly — after around perhaps an hour, or an hour and a half for a first baby. Although the contractions are apparently less intense and less painful in the water, the mother can feel that they are nevertheless more efficient.

The positive effects of immersion in a bath at body temperature are not surprising, in fact, as this is an obvious way to reduce dramatically the level of adrenaline. It is well established — thanks to the works of Regina Lederman in particular — that a low level of adrenaline tends to make the first stage of labor easier and faster. More generally speaking, any experienced birth attendant knows that a situation tending to increase the level of adrenaline — fear, cold, and so forth — makes the first stage more difficult. It is not by chance that such an acute observer as Grantly Dick-Read called his main work *Childbirth without Fear.*

But when the baby is not far away, there comes a time when some mothers feel that the contractions are not working efficiently any longer. After a series of five, or six, or seven contractions, there may be no further progress; and then many women feel the need to get out of the pool. As soon as they leave the warm bath and return to the cooler atmosphere of the room, a puzzling phenomenon often occurs. It is as if a kind of reflex were triggered by the difference of temperature and, after a few huge contractions, the baby is born on the floor by the pool. This, then, is truly a fetus ejection reflex.

The phenomenon is difficult to interpret if you have been imbued with the simplistic idea that every situation in which the level of adrenaline is raised will always tend to slow down the delivery. Indeed, this is a situation when a rush of adrenaline is associated with strong and efficient contractions. Some women even get goose bumps — a well-known sign of the release of the hormone we secrete when we are cold or frightened.

I took the first step toward my interpretation of human birth along the lines of Niles Newton's work with other mammals on the day when I made the connection between an authentic fetus ejection reflex and other situations accompanied by a rush of adrenaline. I remember some deliveries when the baby was born "like a shot out of a gun," after the mother had seemed fearful. Many midwives have told me similar stories. I have been told that, in the past, some French doctors would say something frightening just before deciding to use forceps because they knew that, occasionally, this might be a way to avoid having to use them. And there are documents suggesting that various human groups throughout history have known that a sudden sense of fear can trigger just such a fetus ejection reflex at a very precise stage of the delivery, in very precise circumstances.

The following paragraph is an extract from an eighteenth-century book found in a Paris library, written by a certain J-C. B. after a trip to Canada. It concerns the lifestyle of a tribe of Canadian Indians:

> Women usually give birth by themselves and without any difficulty, and always away from their own homes in small huts which have been built in the forest for this purpose, forty or fifty days beforehand. Sometimes they even give birth in their fields. If it happens — which is rare — that a woman should have a difficult labor, the young people of the village are called and, all of a sudden, when the woman is not expecting anything, they all shout out close to her and the sudden shock triggers the delivery.

This text is evidence that these people had an extremely subtle knowledge of the process of birth. One can imagine that an experienced woman was following the event discreetly from a distance. She knew exactly when the occasion called for an injection of a little adrenaline. Every word is important in this short and concise paragraph. For example, the word *small* regarding the birthing hut is an important detail for anyone who appreciates the meaning of privacy.

These correlations led me to an interpretation of the fetus ejection reflexes observed at births where there has been no interference at all. These really are births according to the method of the mammals. There has been neither a change of environmental temperature, nor any alarming word spoken. Yet, without taking a blood sample and without being an exceptionally acute observer, one can easily guess that there has been a rush of adrenaline during many fast ends of delivery.

During the first stage, most of these women are rather passive—lying on one side, or kneeling on all fours—and seem perfectly self-confident; but suddenly they have enormous muscular energy for the last few contractions. At the end of a home birth in the middle of an authentic fetus ejection reflex, I remember a woman who was grasping my hand with one hand and my shirt with the other. What energy! Then again, some women try to hang onto something or somebody with such tremendous strength that their feet even leave the ground. A sudden need to grasp something and to flex the knees is so typical that it makes any vaginal examination unnecessary. This is the time when many women will not hesitate to take off their clothes, which earlier had protected their privacy. The fetus ejection reflex is usually accompanied by an urgent need to drink some water. A dry mouth is well known as a symptom of adrenaline secretion. Her breathing will be superficial, moving only in the upper part of the chest. The short out-breath is interrupted during the contractions. Her pupils are completely dilated. The powerful contractions at the end are sometimes accompanied by the expression of anger. For example, some women furiously kick at a wall with their elbow or knee. This is another well-known symptom of a rush of adrenaline. Other women suddenly become euphoric—yet another typical symptom of a rush of adrenaline.

What is the factor that triggers this release of adrenaline when the mother experiences neither a change of temperature nor any sense of alarm? I came to attach great importance to a comment made by the German anthropologist Wulf Schiefenhovel when he visited us in Pithiviers. Wulf has a deep understanding and knowledge of a very "primitive" tribe in New Guinea called the Eipos. Some minutes before a rapid end to a delivery, a woman had openly expressed her fear. Wulf noticed it and said, "That's interesting. The Eipos say exactly the same thing at the same time." Two days later, while I was trying to interpret what this mother had felt and expressed, she told me, "I never said that. I wasn't afraid of anything."

This story prompted me to analyze more carefully the short period between the passive phase and the onset of the reflex. I found that — more often than not — just before the expulsive contractions begin, some women express fear in a more or less direct way. It might be, "I am scared. I am going to die." Or, "What's happening?" — said in a tone that suggests fear triggered by a threatening and uncertain situation. Or body language that expresses sudden anxiety, without any word spoken. If during this short phase of transition there is no interference at all — no word to reassure; no comment about the present stage of labor; nobody behaving like an observer — and if the woman can express her fear freely, the strong contractions of the ejection reflex build up suddenly and work as efficiently as possible.

This is how I arrived at the concept of "physiological fear." It is as if, at a certain stage when there is a sudden change in the mother's hormonal balance, a certain degree of fear can be interpreted as a rush of adrenaline, while it would be anger or euphoria for other women. As a matter of fact, many mammals seem to express some kind of anxiety at a certain stage during birth. The concept of physiological fear is difficult for us to accept and assimilate in a world where it is commonplace to classify the emotions as clearly either positive or negative, and to try to cultivate the positive ones and to dispense with the others. But this sort of classification means nothing to physiologists. Any emotion can be seen as a change in the hormonal balance, and it has a specific role to play. In the same way, one has to accept that there is a role to be performed by physiological pain among humans and other mammals during birthing, inasmuch as the secretion of certain kinds of endorphins is necessary for the release of the hormone for lactation — prolactin — which plays a part in completing the maturation of the baby's lungs. And these endorphins might also play a part in the bonding between mother and newborn.

These observations are not at odds with what has been known for a long time through experimental injections of adrenaline during labor. It is just that people only remember from these studies that such injections stop the process of birth, which is true in most cases. But when you read the articles reporting these studies from start to finish, and not just the summaries alone, you realize that the results were in fact contradictory. The injection either triggers the delivery or else inhibits it after some strong contractions. And these observations are not out of line with what we know about the subjective effects of *any* injection of adrenaline. The famous experiments by Schacter–Singer demonstrated that, depending on the context, an injection of adrenaline could induce a state either of euphoria or of anger. In the context of birthing, then, not only is it possible to confirm that in some circumstances a rush of adrenaline can have the paradoxical effect of triggering strong and efficient contractions but, moreover, this paradoxical effect can now be interpreted in the scientific paradigm of the 1990s.[1]

Since we do not hesitate here to consider human beings primarily as mammals, a question immediately comes to mind. What do these findings mean in a natural environment? What is their significance in the jungle? And indeed, these findings do make sense in a natural environment. Imagine that a female in labor is suddenly threatened by a predator. At the beginning of labor, it would be an advantage to interrupt the process, to postpone it, and to put the female in a good physiological state for fighting or running away. On the contrary, once she has passed the point of no return, as it were, it would be an advantage for her to give birth as quickly as possible and then be in a position to fight and protect the offspring.

So, having some experience with unmanaged deliveries in

an atmosphere of perfect privacy, in the dark, with the mother feeling free to be noisy and to adopt any comfortable position, one gets a new vision of the different stages of birth. In the usual context of a modern birth, it is the midwife's or the doctor's finger that gives information about the progress of labor. The complete dilation of the cervix marks the border between first stage and second stage: "Now you are fully dilated — you can push."

When a woman is allowed to give birth according to the method of the mammals, the finger is uncalled for. Many aspects of the mother's behavior — her breathing, the noise she makes, her position — provide the attendant with much more insight. The first stage and second stage are not distinguished by reference to the dilation of the mother's cervix any longer, but according to the way she behaves and her state of consciousness — that is to say, her hormonal balance. Besides, the finger can be misleading. Complete dilation of the cervix can greatly precede the onset of the ejection reflex. This is more frequent in certain ethnic groups, particularly among black African women. Conversely, the ejection reflex can also precede complete dilation. From my own experience, I have found this most frequently among Portuguese and Turkish women.

This gives us an inkling of the extreme complexity of childbirth, the physiology of which has never been seriously studied as far as humans are concerned. In terms of its complexity, the process of birth can be compared with other events in the field of sexual life. For example, birth shares certain points in common with the male orgasm, where the first phase — or phase of erection — is not under the influence of nerves that use adrenaline as a mediator. The second phase, on the other hand — the phase of ejaculation (sperm ejection reflex) — is under the control of sympathetic nerves that do work via the medium of adrenaline. In both cases — childbirth and male orgasm — there is a succession of rather passive phases followed by an active, violent, and even aggressive one.

Let us dream of a time when the art of midwifery will be primarily the practice of not hindering the fetus ejection reflex. Then the post-electronic age will be established. There is no reason why the advent of such an age should be impossible. The appropriate nonintrusive technology is on hand. The symbol of this new era might be the small ultrasound stethoscope, which looks like an electric razor and is usually called a Doptone or small Sonicaid. With this little device, one can now and then evaluate the rhythm of the baby's heartbeat before, during, and after a contraction. It is possible to listen to the baby's heart whatever the mother's position, provided that she is not leaning forward. Since the vaginal exam will become less and less useful, the only remaining excuse that birth attendants will have to disturb the laboring woman will be to listen to the baby with this little device as discreetly and infrequently as possible. Finding the right moment for this examination, and judging how often it should be repeated, are part of the art of midwifery. An experienced midwife takes a great number of criteria into consideration — such as the condition of the amniotic sac, what she knows about the color of the fluid, the behavior of the mother and her level of anxiety, and so on. It becomes unnecessary to listen to the baby's heart tones when the point of no return has obviously been reached and the baby will almost certainly be born within ten minutes. Auscultation, like any other interference, is dangerous when the ejection reflex is about to start, as it might inhibit it and make the birth much longer. Anyway, interference — whether a vaginal exam or even an auscultation — is almost impossible in the middle of an authentic fetus ejection reflex.

Although the incidence of babies becoming distressed during labor will decrease with the advent of this new era, we should not ever lose the ability to detect babies in difficulty. Should the method of the mammals be inefficient in any particular instance, there must always be teams capable of doing epidurals to compensate for the lack of endorphins; to use drips to compensate for a deficiency of hormones from the posterior pituitary; and to perform cesarean sections to rescue babies in distress.

In fact, technology is ready for the advent of the post-electronic age, but people are not. We cannot replace obstetrics — a discipline whose priority is to control childbirth — with a radically new attitude whose priority would be to make birth as easy as possible, and expect to do it overnight.

The kind of research some obstetricians are conducting is symptomatic of a deep misunderstanding of the physiological processes of birth, and of a strong need to control them. We are still at a stage where researchers are looking into which is the best birthing position. Groups of women are allocated, at random, to adopt this or that position. From the experience of women who did not feel observed when giving birth and felt as free as possible, I have come to understand that it is not the position itself that matters; it is the mother's hormonal balance. But her hormonal balance will influence her posture. When the level of adrenaline is low, the tendency is to lie down and keep still. If there is a rush of adrenaline, one tends to be upright. During a fetus ejection reflex, it is not the upright position that is important, however, but the tendency or need to be upright. At the onset of the last contractions, the best position is usually the one that nobody has foreseen.

When you are familiar with births culminating in an authentic fetus ejection reflex, your approach is quite unorthodox in every stage of labor. For example, the attitude regarding the perineum is unusual. The mother will often be standing up during the last contractions, bending forward, leaning on the edge of a piece of furniture, or feeling the need to hang onto something; or else she is on all fours, and things are going fast. Either way, you only need to hold out your hand so that the baby does not fall on the floor. You lose the habit of looking at the perineum, and touching it. An episiotomy is out of the question. And besides, serious tearing is a very rare occurrence following a real ejection reflex. This observation leads us to a number of complementary interpretations. In the first place, the contractions are not inhibited by a self-styled expert giving orders about when to push, whether to push this way or that way, or how to breathe in this fashion or that. It is well known that when deliveries are spontaneous and unmanaged, such as sometimes occur in elevators or corridors, serious tears are rare. Most women instinctively adopt a position during the last contractions such that the vulva can distend more evenly. I have found that tears are unusual when the mother-to-be is bending forward during the last contractions. She might be standing up and leaning forward over the edge of a table, or on all fours. When she is hanging onto something or somebody, or when her shoulders are supported from beneath, there is an upward force that balances the force going down. At the same time the muscles of the thighs relax completely — especially the inner thighs, where the muscles coordinate their action with the muscles of the perineum. When these muscles are able to relax, it is as if a door were opening; when they are prevented from relaxing, the door must be forced. It is not by chance that, in Latin, they are called *custodes virginatis* (the guardians of the virginity).

Moreover, when an ejection reflex occurs, it is usually quite unnecessary to assist the delivery of the baby's shoulders with your hands. Tears often happen at that time. If help is really essential because the baby is very large, it is better to wait after the delivery of the head, and do nothing; then, at the peak of the next contraction, intervene if necessary, but be as gentle and efficient as possible.

The need for privacy does not end when the baby is born. An environment that enhances the delivery is also needed immediately afterward, so as not to disturb the first contact between mother and baby. Quite often, if the mother is not inhibited from doing so, she first touches the baby's body timidly with her fingertips and then, as she gets more and more confident, dares to take it up in her arms. This is the time of the first skin-to-skin and eye-to-eye contact. It is as if the eyes of the mother were attracted by the baby's eyes, and vice versa. Methodical studies have demonstrated that the human newborn is programed to direct its gaze toward everything that resembles a pair of eyes distanced about a foot away from its own face. This eye-to-eye contact seems to be a crucial moment in the mother-baby relationship. But there is almost always somebody around who wants to disturb it, either clumsily or in a more subtle way. This is the most difficult time to protect the atmosphere of privacy. Few fathers manage to be discreet or respectful of what is basically a one-to-one relationship. But only if this one-to-one relationship is not interrupted by the activity of people around can the baby's first suckling take place in the hour following birth — which, incidentally, helps to keep the blood loss accompanying the detachment of the placenta to a minimum. The best way to avoid hemorrhage is to enable mother and baby to stay in close contact in a warm, dark, and silent place — and get rid of any observers. The contact with the baby's eyes and skin helps the mother to secrete the hormone necessary to stimulate the "placenta ejection reflex." When the baby suckles the nipple, the reflex is reinforced.

Interestingly, when the mother feels uninhibited and is not given any orders, or even any suggestions, she tends of her own accord to find a position that minimizes compression of the big vein returning blood from the uterus to the heart; and in so doing, she reduces her own blood loss. (For, as everybody has probably observed, if you want to make a vein bleed a little more—for example, in taking a blood sample—you just have to compress the flow downstream.)

The mother might be sitting on the floor, bending forward slightly as she holds the baby in her arms, or lying down on one side, with the baby close to her body. Anyhow, there is no compression of the big vein called the *vena cava*. Just as during the delivery itself, in this postdelivery stage it is out of the question to recommend one good position in particular. In fact there is only one positively bad position: the mother lying on her back but semiseated, with the baby on her tummy. In this position, the weight of the baby plus the weight of the uterus will tend to compress the vena cava. Yet this is the situation always created or at least encouraged by attendants, and it usually follows a delivery accomplished with the mother reclining on her back—which happens very rarely when there has been an authentic fetus ejection reflex.

The mother often remains active after such a reflex, alert and upright for some minutes. It is as if the effects of the rush of adrenaline were continuing after the birth. After a while though—often five to ten minutes—many mothers need to lie down. It is probable that the excess of adrenaline has been eliminated.[2] Often at this time the mother will complain of feeling cold. The room temperature should be very warm—even hot—for the mother and the baby. A lying-down position might also, at this point, be a way to reduce blood loss.

It is because a few simple principles are not understood that the fear of hemorrhage after birth remains so strong. Some academic studies have led to incredible results. For example, in one British hospital the obstetric staff found that, if they did not use a certain drug to stimulate the delivery of the placenta and did not cut the cord and pull it, the risk of hemorrhage was 17 percent! If the risk were even 1 percent, I should not dare to assist home births and I would not accept any woman for a home birth who had suffered a hemorrhage after a previous birth in a hospital. But in fact, I am so convinced that most hemorrhages are due to an improper environment that I *have* accepted such a case.

Whatever the stage of labor, and whatever the type of birth, these few simple principles can be brought to bear so long as the importance of privacy is held paramount. Perhaps they are still more important when you are expecting a difficulty. For example, you have no fear of a breech birth when you know how to eliminate all the factors that might get in the way of the fetus ejection reflex. Of course, you will have to do a cesarean section if the first stage is long and difficult in spite of the mother's enjoying complete privacy. But in most cases a vaginal birth is possible and, thanks to the reflex and the use of upright postures, you should not have to pull the baby out. I would not approach the risk of a breech birth by allocating this or that position. In the same way, it would be dangerous to disturb the physiological processes in the case of a low-weight baby, a vaginal birth after cesarean, or a first baby born to a mother over forty.

Whatever the mother's medical background, her birthing needs for dim lighting, a familiar place, and the absence of observers are now more important than ever.

Notes

1. A rush of adrenaline tends to trigger a release of free fatty acids by destroying the lipids. When there is a nonselective release of free fatty acids, the dominant one — that is, the most abundant — is the direct precursor (in this case, arachidonic acid) of the different prostaglandins involved in the birth process. The phenomena involved in this process are fast and transitory. Also, adrenaline acts via two kinds of uterine receptors. The beta-receptors are inhibitory, while the alpha-receptors are excitatory. Below a certain threshold, only the beta-receptors might be activated, while above a certain threshold (when there is a rush of

adrenaline), the alpha receptors are involved. The ratio between alpha and beta tends to increase at the end of pregnancy. This is probably one reason why an authentic fetus ejection reflex is rare in the case of a premature birth, while it is common in the case of a birth at term of a small-for-dates baby.

2. These observations are in agreement with the work of Regina Lederman. She found that adrenaline values return to normal within three to twenty-one minutes after delivery.

CHAPTER SIX

Cats

Iona called me one afternoon as contractions forewarned her of the beginning of labor. Even before knocking at the door, I was intrigued by the noise of a vacuum cleaner. Between contractions, Iona was "hoovering." During contractions, she was leaning on the back of a chair. I asked her afterward if she usually did the cleaning in the middle of the afternoon. "What?! No!" she said. "I don't know what made me do that today." Such behavior goes unnoticed by anyone ignorant of our mammalian condition. Or if it is noticed, it is incomprehensible.

In fact, Iona's vacuuming was simply one manifestation of the "nesting instinct." This instinct is by no means exclusive to birds and insects who build nests. It is the behavior that drives the animal to prepare, in one way or another, the space in which it will welcome its offspring. There are even some mammals, such as the dormouse, who actually build nests.

My experience of home birth is based to a large extent on the recognition of this nesting instinct. In modern cities, most pregnant women choose the place of birth as early as the first months of pregnancy. They usually book themselves into a hospital. But sometimes a woman will suddenly develop "hospital phobia," often two or three weeks before the birth. In most cases she does not dare to express this phobia openly, or even her reluctance about going into the hospital. And if she does try to explain it in words, those around her are quick to persuade her to return to a more "reasonable" attitude.

But occasionally the mother-to-be decides to stay at home, against all odds. Of course, she avoids discussing this with her doctor, anticipating his first question: "And what will you do if something goes wrong?" She contacts other people whom she knows will be more sympathetic to her feelings.

I have learned a lot from women in this situation who have managed to get in touch with me via word of mouth. Their behavior is incomprehensible to doctors whose only horizon is an obstetric hospital service, to many administrative personnel, and to anyone and everyone who ignore the fact that we humans are mammals. These people want to know why. While there are places — they ask — where everything is provided for the safety of birth, with qualified staff, specialized machinery, and surgical equipment, why on Earth do pregnant women want to stay at home? "These women must be out of their minds!"

Christine did not want to go to the hospital for the birth of her first baby. She succumbed under pressure from serious and experienced people. In the end she had a cesarean. For the second baby, she listened first of all to her own feelings. She had a straightforward three-hour labor at home in the middle of the night. I was asleep in the next room and was awakened by the characteristic cry of the ejection reflex. Christine had alerted me earlier in the night when she felt some preliminary symptoms. In an atmosphere of self-confidence, complete privacy, and safety, the contractions were extremely efficient. This is a common occurrence and one that can be foreseen. I always prefer to get settled in as soon as the very first symptoms appear. When I visit a woman who is planning a home birth, she usually asks me what to prepare. One of my answers is "A bed for me." It might be a sofa or a mattress on the floor, but that's fine. Once I have my own territory — a place where I can read or sleep — the privacy of the future mother is assured at the same time. Of course, this is not my only answer to a mother's practical questions. I talk first about heating, and the importance of having an extra mobile heater capable of working quickly anywhere at any time, even in the middle of July and in the best heated apartments. It is important during a birth that the mother feels as comfortable as possible in terms of temperature. And while it is always easy to open a window if it gets too hot, it can be more difficult to deal with a sudden feeling of cold. This is especially important just after the birth. Then, more often than not, the place has to be much warmer than usual. When the new mother starts shaking, it is not physiological; it is because she is not warm enough. The right temperature is an important factor in facilitating the detachment of the placenta. The newborn, too, has a great need for warmth. Even if the temperature of the room is high, it is usually a good idea to cover the infant's back with a warm towel.

At the time of birth especially, we should not forget that Man was originally a tropical mammal. Then too, the nesting instinct in our species also implies the protection of the baby in terms of heat. It is easier to interpret certain statistics when you take the human nesting instinct into account. Thus, Holland has the best statistics in the world at the present time, if one considers that it is the only country with a perinatal mortality rate below 10 per 1,000, a maternal mortality rate below 1 per 10,000, and a cesarean rate in the region of 6 percent. It is also the only highly industrialized country where one baby in three is born at home, one in three is born in a maternity unit (that is, in a hospital with a midwife who is not under the control of an obstetrician), and only one in three in a conventional obstetric unit. In other words, the nesting instinct can express itself more effectively at home than anywhere else. When obstetrics becomes more genuinely scientific, no one will hesitate to look these statistics squarely in the face and it will be easier for people to understand that opting for home birth in modern urban society is not a step back into the past.

A good understanding of the nesting instinct would have many practical implications. Thus, for administrative reasons women are often pressured into making choices as early as possible during their pregnancy. They have to decide where they are going to have their baby. But there is some danger in making these choices prematurely. The choice is then made intellectually and rationally. But in order to have due regard for the instinctive forces that tend to express themselves only at the end of pregnancy, it would be more beneficial for women to keep several options open and to postpone a final decision.

One cannot acquire a profound knowledge, or rather an understanding of the whole period surrounding birth, without having experience of home birth. The "school of home birth" has trained few pupils during the past few decades. But these very pupils will have a significant role to play in laying the foundations of the post-electronic era. One of their roles will naturally be to integrate home birth into modern society. Another will be to design the birthing centers of tomorrow, situating them in close proximity with hospital facilities, and training staff members who will increasingly take on the role previously played by the extended family in the home. In addition, those experienced in home birth will play a part in designing obstetric services intended for mothers and babies who do require medical help.

Every hospital in the world tends to make the same mistakes. Let us take the example of the beds found in maternity wards. They are usually high and narrow. For this reason, mothers do not dare to have their babies sleep with them, in case they should fall out. Thus, the time for skin-to-skin contact is reduced, and the start of breastfeeding is made more difficult. Experience with home births has shown me that many young couples now have low, wide beds. There is no fear of falling out of them, and the mother does not hesitate to sleep with her baby. This is just one example suggesting that the school of home birth can help us to acquire a vision of the way hospitals should be in the future. I have now reached the point where I find it difficult to tolerate the environment of a hospital, even though I spent thirty-five years of my working life there.

The experience of home birth can also be a source of knowledge that *cannot* be applied elsewhere. For example, I learnt a great deal about cats. Is there a correlation between the presence of cats in a house and a fast birth? Years ago such a question would not have occurred to me. Nevertheless, evidence gathered by my own eyes now tells me there is such a correlation. This leads to another question. Given that such a correlation does exist, could it be that a love for cats and the capacity to give birth easily are two aspects of the same kind of temperament? To be a cat lover can signify a love of calm, a love of caressing in a certain way, a love of giving to those who ask, and to those on whom one cannot, in turn, make demands. This may coincide with the capacity to surrender to the animal side of one's behavior and to allow oneself to be dominated by life events. Or, alternatively, does living with cats tend to shape the personality? Do cats bring to our daily lives enough calm, serenity, and detachment to regulate the levels of stress hormones among those around them? Or, indeed, could it be that cats are endowed with a mysterious power? Is it possible that they can directly influence the course of labor simply by their presence? We should not forget that the Egyptians worshiped cats as sacred animals and even mummified their dead bodies. In fact, one cemetery containing more than 300 cats has been discovered! As a sign of mourning for a beloved fe-line, the Egyptians used to shave their eyebrows. And to kill a cat was to risk the death penalty. Furthermore, Bestel, the goddess of love and fertility, had the head of a cat and the body of a woman. Could it be that cats have "bioenergetic" properties we are unable to identify and explain? Cats have the reputation of being endowed with metaphysical powers. What are the bases for this belief?

One London therapist allows her cats to come and go in her consulting room. She has observed that they are at-tracted by pregnant women and in particular by their bel-lies. Some clairvoyants claim to need the presence of a cat to reinforce their powers of prediction. It has also been noticed that cats are drawn toward some people more than others, and that they like to lie on certain parts of the body such as the stomach and the neck. These parts of the body corre-spond exactly to two of the chakras, the subtle energy cen-ters described by the Initiates of India — centers that are said to be totally active only in a minority of human beings, and that only yogis know how to stimulate consciously.

Cats are indeed mysterious from many points of view. It seems that their behavior is not affected in the same way as dogs by telluric and electromagnetic influences. Some ob-servers claim that a cat tends to occupy disturbed zones and, as such, can reestablish the equilibrium, playing the role of regulator or even protector. A dog, on the other hand, would behave differently, more like a human being.

In any case, the curious relationship between cats and pregnant women seems to have been recognized throughout the ages. Why did the great painters of the past introduce the cat as a typical component in their representations of the scene of the Annunciation?

Or is it not rather that cats have a special relationship with pregnant mammals in general? This question is raised in "Midwife Cat," a poem by Mark van Doren.

Till at the threshold of a shed
She smells the water and the corn
Where a sow is on her bed
And little pigs are being born.

Silently she leaps, and walks
All night upon a narrow rafter,
Whence at intervals she talks
Wise to them she watches after.

It is indeed tempting to propose a comparison between the effect of cats on labor and that of water or of an authentic midwife. We should not forget that for some psychoanalysts the cat is, above all, a feminine symbol. Carl Jung—in his studies of dreams and his interpretation of the genesis of mental illness—saw the cat as an erotic symbol.

This brings us to Igor Tcharkovsky, the sea, and dolphins. Tcharkovsky claims that dolphins can communicate with human babies in the womb in a mysterious way described, at present, as telepathic, and can help them to get rid of a potential fear of water. He dreams of a world where pregnant women swim with dolphins and give birth in their company. For the majority of people, this new kind of mutual help between species belongs to the realm of fantasy or utopia, even though some do acknowledge that communication via meditation may very well be possible.

Why should we not first try to confirm whether or not our familiar domestic animals have some influence on the birth of human babies and, if they do, analyze this influence? This might have some very practical implications. If a love of cats turns out to be the important factor in the cat-pregnancy connection, this might give a new significance to (and change a few attitudes about) baby girls and cats living together. (Some people would also stress that this would, at the same time, be a good way for girls to become immune to toxoplasmosis—a disease that can be transmitted by cats, but that in practice is dangerous only for babies in the womb.) Or if it is the presence itself of the animal that is important, this would no doubt encourage a number of women to stay at home to give birth. But it would certainly require a major shift in awareness for such factors to be taken into consideration at the teaching hospitals!

If my attention has been drawn to cats rather than dogs or other domestic animals, it is because they behave in a particularly exemplary way during a birth. They are as discreet as possible. You do not see them, but they are there. In spite of their apparent indifference, they seem to know exactly what is going on, sensing the importance and even the sanctity of the event.

The behavior of cats during labor could be a source of inspiration for midwives of the future. To escape notice while, at the same time, being able to detect if something is wrong—this just about sums up the art of midwifery. It must involve the deepest aspects of the personality. Not many people are endowed with the capacity to remain unnoticed.

Gender has to be taken into consideration. In the birthing place, a woman—especially one who has had children herself and is not enmeshed in a web of fear—will be less conspicuous than a man. This does not mean that a woman who has not had children cannot fulfil the role of midwife. The laboring woman needs a particular kind of privacy, however. At a certain stage of labor, she has to open her sphincters and empty the rectum. At this point she needs the type of privacy that is not disturbed by a mother, or a woman who brings to mind a mother or a grandmother. On the other hand, the presence of a sexual partner can be inhibiting. Also, a more mature person will be less conspicuous than someone younger. In many languages, the word for "midwife" (for example, in French *matrone* and *sage-femme*) evokes wisdom acquired through age and experience. In America, the midwife is traditionally called "a grannie."

The capacity to escape notice is also a matter of education and training, and even of technique. Performing very few vaginal examinations, or none at all, is one way of being discreet. I have some tapes that might be useful for the training of the midwives of tomorrow. From an adjoining room one can, with sufficient experience, nearly always evaluate the progress of labor simply by listening. And as mentioned in Chapter 5, the small ultrasound stethoscope of the Doptone or Sonicaid type does not require the woman to lie down for the baby's heartbeat to be heard before, during, and after a contraction. This small gadget could take on the dimensions of a technological breakthrough — for those who can behave like cats.

CHAPTER SEVEN

The Old and the New

For many primitive peoples the origin of life is a sound: it
is the voice of God. . . . Why primitive peoples should believe this may be implicit in the cry of the newborn babe
who, separated from the mother as he struggles into an
alien world, yells for mammalian security.
                    —Wilfrid Mellers, *Bach and the Dance of God*

Human beings are condemned to live with two brains.
Whatever approach one might take toward apprehending
the human phenomenon, it must always take into consideration some aspect of the relationship between our two
brains — the old one and the new one.

Sexual Events

We have seen that the activity of the primitive brain pre-
vails during the process of birth. We share this primitive or
archaic brain with all the mammals. It is old also in the
sense that it reaches maturity very early on in our lives, at
the age when we are still dependent on our mothers. It cannot be dissociated from the hormonal system and the im-

mune system, with which it forms a complex network. This
network itself represents the adaptive systems involved in
what we commonly call "health." The archaic brain, which
governs the emotions and instincts, can also be looked on as
a gland releasing the hormones necessary for the process of
birth, inducing efficient uterine contractions, and protect-
ing against pain as well.

The process of birth is all the easier when the other brain,
the new brain, takes a backseat. This new brain—the neocortex, whose huge development is the main feature of human beings—does not reach maturity before adulthood. Its
activity during the process of birth only hinders the activity
of the old brain. All inhibitions come from the neocortex
during a delivery (and in any other event of the sexual life,
as well). That is why, in a very spontaneous birth according
to the method of the mammals, there is a stage when the
woman seems to be cut off from our world, as if on her way
to another planet. This changing level of consciousness is
obviously related to a lesser degree of control by the new
brain. Then the mother-to-be is freed from any sort of inhibition. She dares to scream out; to open her sphincters; to
forget about what she has learned, what is cultural, even
what is decent. That is why the best way to make a birth
longer, more difficult, more painful (and more dangerous)
is to stimulate the neocortex where all the inhibitions origi-
nate.

The neocortex can be stimulated by light, or by having to
listen to people talking logically and rationally, or by being
surrounded by people who behave like observers. A feeling
of privacy, on the other hand, accompanies a reduction in
neocortical control.

It cannot be emphasized enough that the active part of
the brain during a delivery and other events of the sexual
life is that which develops early in the life of each individual—during a period I have called "the primal period"—
and which encompasses the life in the womb, the period

around birth and early infancy. Focusing on this early development leads one to suspect that any serious preparation for birth (or for sexual life) should concentrate on this period!

Thus, in our study of the relationship between "the old and the new," we start by considering the primary behavior essential for the survival of the species: sexual activity, and in particular the process of birth. We have seen how these activities can be repressed, inhibited by the new brain. So we shall point out the distinction between Homo sapiens and the other mammals. Homo sapiens is the only mammal whose neocortex is strong enough to inhibit, to repress, and even to threaten the instincts that are indispensable for the survival of the species.[1] On the one hand, the neocortex is a tool at the service of the brain that supports the dynamics of survival. On the other hand, it exceeds its role as a tool, and often seems to be interfering in activities that are much too complex for its abilities and negligent of its original assignment. Hence the conflict.

The processes of inhibition can work both ways, however. The old brain — the emotional one — can, sometimes, inhibit the rational brain. We all know that a strong emotion can make us lose our capacity for logical reasoning. Think of the candidate for an exam who is paralyzed by fear, unable to resolve an equation he would find easy in other circumstances.

The Gap between Two Kinds of Knowledge

It is as if the two levels were storing different and incompatible sorts of knowledge. The new brain, which makes a scientific attitude possible, supports the concepts of time, space, and boundaries, including the limit of our own lifespan. It gives us a sense of our identity, which, together with a sense of our limits in space, is only reached it seems when the human neocortex has developed to a certain degree, corresponding to the stage when the child can recognize himself or herself in a mirror. The concept of limits in time leads to the knowledge of death.

The old structures, on the other hand, contain the knowledge that we are part of a whole. They support the religious sense, which transcends the concepts of space and time. Insofar as the old brain also engenders the will to survive, the universal religious sense will go on expressing itself as long as there are humans who struggle for life. It is part of human nature.

It is significant that, at a certain stage of labor, many women express a fear of death. Beyond that stage, their fear seems to have been overcome. Then the delivery can quickly come to an end with an authentic fetus ejection reflex. It is as if the knowledge and the fear of death, which are contained in the new brain, tend to vanish when a particular state of consciousness is reached. It is as if the woman in labor had a physiological mechanism at her disposal so that, at the right moment, she can forget this knowledge and fear that are characteristic features of our species. And this physiological mechanism is the reduction in control exercised by the new brain.

From a scientific viewpoint, real knowledge is stored in the neocortex. From the Buddhist point of view, or that of a mystic, real knowledge is obtained only by meditation, by getting rid of the whirl of sensory stimuli and ideas that constantly distract us. The gap between the knowledge retained in our two brains is the reason for philosophy. Any work or any school of philosophy cannot be dissociated from a given period of history, because it makes reference to scientific knowledge that is itself subject to change.

Not only do the two brains contain different sorts of knowledge, but they also have different needs. How is it possible to reconcile scientific curiosity with the need for the irrational, magic, superstition, and with the need to believe in something? Well, as a matter of fact, it is not beyond a scientific approach to explain how faith — which satisfies the needs of the old brain — can influence the workings of the most primitive adaptive systems, that is, health. In other words, modern science can explain how faith will save you.

This example suggests that the conflict between our two brains does not mean they are completely divorced. The opposition between the old brain and the new brain as described here is deliberately simplistic. Modern physiology suggests that the right side of the neocortex has a closer relation with the old brain than the left side, and that there might be a difference in this according to gender. Besides, there are situations when the activities of both brains harmonize, complement, and even reinforce each other. One fitting instance of this harmony can be seen in the function of singing.

The Function of Singing

Let us go back to those birthing places, to those maternity hospitals or birthing centers, where women can meet to sing (see Chapter 3). Singing is a specifically human activity. And the need for a resurgence of fundamental humanity is strong during pregnancy. There is no example of a human society where singing was unknown. Thus, anyone who would study what makes Man special in the world of mammals should certainly reflect on the function of singing. I grew to understand this over time, after singing with pregnant women in France, the United Kingdom, and the United States.

A birthing center or a maternity hospital is an ideal place to realize that the voice can be at the service of the most primitive brain structures. This is so in the case of the scream that characterizes the last contraction before birth, and also the first cry of the newborn baby. As a matter of fact, similar vocalizations have been reproduced in animal experiments by stimulating very precise areas of the primitive brain with electrodes. But when a pregnant woman asks her doctor if her level of Anti-D antibodies has increased since the previous visit, she is putting her voice at the service of the most recent layers of her neocortex. Finally, when singing, the voice is at the service of the primitive brain and the new brain (which makes language possible) at the same time. The direct communication of emotions through melody and rhythm is completed by the use of words. Among human beings endowed with the capacity to speak, singing is a perfect example of how both brains can work in harmony.

This can be said of the whole breathing function, as well — without which there would be no vocal function. Breathing is usually under the control of very primitive nervous structures. We breathe without thinking about it. But the neocortex can assume breathing movements. It can suddenly decide to breathe quickly and superficially. When we sing, the two brains manage to harmonize their powers of control.

Studying the function of singing is a key to understanding human beings. In fact, in any artistic activity, a technique — which is governed by the specifically human neocortex — puts itself at the service of a function controlled by older structures. The technique of a musician makes it possible to transmit emotions through sound. The technique of a painter can transmit emotions with visual signals. Poetry is the transmission of emotions via our elaborate form of communication called "language." The technique of a dancer tends to arouse emotions induced by body movements and rhythms. Gastronomy is related to digestive functions; the art of the perfume maker, to the sense of smell; eroticism, to the mating instinct. There is no physiological function that cannot be the basis for artistic activity. It is significant that words like "art" and "artifice" have the same root. Indeed, art is an artifice used by humans to harmonize their two brains.

Man and Water

Humans have always tried to bridge the divide — the dichotomy between reason on the one hand, and emotion, faith, passion on the other. Moreover, they have always sought mediators to facilitate this effort; and water seems to have been recognized as the ideal mediator, anywhere and at any time.

All religions, all the healing arts have taken advantage of the power of water — from the sacred springs of ancient traditions, to the baptism of Christ in the River Jordan; from the rites of Aesculapius, to modern thalassotherapy. The fundamental disease of mankind is its exaggerated submission of the primitive brain to the neocortex. This is why religion and medicine cannot be dissociated. In healing a human being, whether we work to release his or her religious sense or whether we try to harmonize his or her two brains is much the same thing.

Just as it was in a birth place that I first understood the function of singing, it was in the same context that I became aware of the power of water on human beings. When in labor, many women have an irresistible attraction to water. They want to take a shower. They want to have a bath. For some laboring women, water seems to help them to escape, to cut themselves off from our world. Mothers-to-be are attracted to maternity hospitals where there are small pools available during birth. In some cities such as London, they can rent transportable pools especially designed for home birth. As we said in Chapter 5, women tend to relax in water during the stage of the dilation of the cervix, and it seems to make their labor shorter and less painful. Indeed, immersion in water at body temperature can have spectacular effects (so long as the laboring woman does not get into the bath too soon). And in some cases, an interesting further phenomenon can be observed: it is as if suddenly, at a certain stage of the delivery when the mother has reached a very special state of consciousness, forgotten everything she has learnt, all the things she has heard or read, she realizes that her baby can be born underwater. Yes, in fact, the birth of a human baby underwater is quite possible.

There are other ways to discover that Man is an aquatic primate. What do people do on vacation? They lie on a beach and look at the waves. Where do they go on a honeymoon? To Venice, or Niagara Falls, or Hawaii.

When interpreting this power of water on Man, one naturally thinks first of life in the womb, in the amniotic fluid. Our primitive brain develops during an aquatic phase of life. But this does not explain the special attraction of water for humans compared with their closest cousins the apes, chimpanzees, gorillas, and orangutans. They also had an aquatic prenatal life, but yet they do not like water. How can we explain this difference? For one thing, we must give credit to the theory about the emergence of Man expressed in 1960 by Sir Alister Hardy of Oxford University. This theory takes into account the fact that a part of the African continent, and in particular the Afar triangle, was probably covered by the sea at a time that might correspond to the "missing link" in the origin of our species. Every feature that makes Man an exception among the apes can be interpreted as a sign of adaptation to water, or as a feature held in common with the sea mammals. According to this thesis, the spectacular development of our neocortex occurred during this phase of adaptation to marine life. Konrad Lorenz had already established as a rule that aquatic animals have bigger skulls — and therefore bigger brains — than their terrestrial cousins. The brain is bigger, for example, in the otter than in the stoat. The swimming monkey of Gabon, the talapoin, is sometimes called "the Buddhist monk" because its brain case is very large in comparison with its body weight. Moreover, only dolphins and whales have reached a degree of brain development comparable with that of humans. One of the most plausible explanations is that the sea contains huge quantities of minerals, long-chain unsaturated fatty acids,[2] and other nutrients that enhance brain development.

When we take this hypothesis into consideration, we are assuming that both of our brains might have developed in water. First, the primitive brain developed mostly inside the uterus—that is to say, in water. Second, the neocortex might have reached its huge development during an aquatic phase of our evolution. In other words, a liquid milieu might have been imprinted deeply on our individual memory in one respect, and on our collective memory as a species in another respect. Then it's no wonder that water is the typical mediator between our two brains!

By being born in a stable, Christ recalled our mammalian nature. But it was only after his baptism in the River Jordan that he could claim, "If you can make One—from two—you'll be the Son of Man."

What Is Health?

The word *health* has never been defined satisfactorily, where humans are concerned. Once more, the best way to advance our understanding in this regard is to take into account the coexistence of the two brains.

The medical definition considers health to be the absence of disease. Rather than being an official definition, this is the understanding of health that is implicitly transmitted via medical vocabulary and medical attitudes. This understanding of the word *health* should be set aside, however. It is, after all, thanks to good health that one can face an attack by virulent microbes, for example, and be victorious at the end of a struggle—in other words, of being ill, with all the typical symptoms. Disease can thus be the expression of good health.

Health is how well our adaptive systems work. But not all our adaptive systems. Which ones, then, are involved in what we commonly call health? An apposite answer to this question will be impossible so long as the brain is studied as a whole and the hormonal system is particularized — and the immune system too.

Common sense immediately tells us which adaptive systems belong to the field of health, and which are outside it. When I put my watch forward an hour at the beginning of summertime, my capacity for adaptation is set into action. But does it belong to the field of health? No. Why? When, on the other hand, I cope with a sudden change of temperature, I use adaptive systems that *do* belong to the field of health. Why? Study in the same way any number of examples and you will find that the common denominator among the adaptive systems involved in what we call health is their development very early in the life of the individual; they reach maturity at the age when the baby becomes a child.

Health is therefore a matter of how well our oldest adaptive systems work — those that were the first to mature. The old brain is directly involved in what we call health, but not the new one. To understand the meaning of the word *health*, once more we have to distinguish between the old brain and the new one, and also do away with the barriers that have been artificially introduced between the old brain, the hormonal system, and the immune system. This is all but one network, inside which information is constantly circulating. How can we possibly still be trying to separate out a hormonal system and a nervous system, inasmuch as the old brain is primarily a gland? How can we possibly treat the immune system idiosyncratically when cells that were once considered to be specific to this system — like lymphocytes — are now better understood. We know now that their membranes can secrete hormones as well as receive hormonal messages. They can also secrete the same chemical mediators as the nerve cells, and be sensitive to their messages.

This new definition enables us to focus on the beginning of life, on the period during which the "primal adaptive system" is reaching maturity. It helps us to understand that all the events occurring during the primal period—that is to say, between conception and the end of infancy—can influence the maturation of the old brain and the other adaptive systems involved in what is called health.

The basic behaviors capable of modulating health in a positive or negative way are also deeply rooted and obviously related to very old structures of the primitive brain. We have come to realize that a state of submission is the typical situation in which illness is created. This is exactly what happens when, facing a threat, one finds it impossible either to fight or to flee. One can only submit. When rats are given electric shocks, they do not get ill because of the electric shocks, but because they are unable to fight or to escape at the time of the shock. Any submissive state triggers a release of hormones such as cortisol, whose prolonged effect is a kind of physiological suicide. Some metabolic pathways are especially vulnerable to this process; and therefore, certain imbalances are characteristic of submission—in particular, the imbalance among those cell regulators called prostaglandins. When a newborn baby in a nursery learns that it is useless to cry, to express its needs, it is already experiencing a state of submission. The defense mechanisms *against* pathogenic situations are also deeply rooted. Anger is one of these mechanisms. Through animal experiments, we know how to trigger anger by stimulating a very primitive part of the old brain. It is interesting to observe that the attacks thus stimulated tend to be directed toward dominating animals. Anger is a healthy reaction that counteracts the negative effects of a submissive situation. It is very primitive behavior. Everybody knows that a twelve-month-old child can express very real anger. He (or she) can also search for substitutes if his basic needs are not met. This is the meaning of the so-called transitional object, such as the old and dirty cloth or blanket to which a child can be so strongly attached.

Therefore, just as we found when studying birth and other episodes of sexual life, when realizing the function of singing and the arts in general, and when investigating the nature of the religious sense and the power of water, so too we see that any modern definition of the word *health* must also take our double brain into consideration.

The Ecological Man

At the end of this twentieth century, any question, any topic for study, any interpretation of human phenomena must be placed within the context of a biosphere in danger. Human mammals should be studied first as powerful agents of desertification, as superpredators. Our capacity to annihilate entire forms of life gives us a special place in the living world, to say the least.

Since ecological science has now led to ecological awareness, many people are beginning to wonder how we might stop destroying the planet. Some have invested all their hopes into developing an appropriate technology, an ecological technology. Others stake everything on a more ecological society. Others have introduced the concepts of ecological philosophy and ecological humanism. I have claimed that our priority should be the genesis of a different Man, "the genesis of an ecological Man" — a species of men and women who have a positive attitude toward life.

Anyone who has a good knowledge of very young children knows that our attitudes toward life become deeply rooted and imprinted in our personalities at a relatively early age. Maria Montessori told the significant story of a two-year-old Hindu child who was looking down at the ground, on which he seemed to be tracing a line with his finger. There was an ant there that had lost two legs and could walk only with difficulty. The child was trying to be helpful by making a track for it. Another child approached; he saw the ant, put his foot out, and crushed it. Through this story, Montessori wanted to demonstrate that a positive attitude toward life can already be destroyed at the age of two. Comparative studies of different cultures suggest that certain human groups have known how to protect a kind of ecological instinct. For example, the Pygmies used to say, "Never cut a tree." It is significant that the cultures having the greatest respect for life, for Mother Earth — such as the Maoris, the Pygmies, the Huichols — are also those that disturb the mother-baby relationship as little as possible. A Pygmy baby is often breastfed for more than five years; and during the night, its only blanket is its mother. In other words, the relationship of humans with Mother Earth seems closely linked with the mother-baby relationship. A study of the connection between Man and the Earth can no longer be dissociated from a study of the attachment between baby and mother. All those who have studied this process of attachment in a scientific way have focused on the concepts of "critical periods," of "sensitive periods" — short periods of time that often follow not long after birth, and that never happen again. These concepts are emphasized in the work of the so-called ethnologists who, following pioneers such as Konrad Lorenz, observe animal and human behavior. They are also confirmed by those who study the hormonal basis of the process of attachment, including the role of the natural opiates — the endorphins — with their property of inducing habits, dependencies. This system of endorphins probably plays an important part in the period right around birth.

Therefore it seems that the important periods — called sensitive or critical — when the mother-child attachment can be either weakened or strengthened correspond with the time when the primitive brain is still developing. When we claim that the attitude toward life is a deeply ingrained characteristic, recognizable at the age of two, we are attaching great importance to the period when the brain we share with all the other mammals is developing. This is the period of dependency on the mother. A positive attitude toward life seems to go hand in hand with the undisturbed development of a strong primitive brain.

Of course, the ecological Man will also be a scientist. Ecology — the study of the relationships among plants, animals, and their environment — is first and foremost a science. Thus, it concerns our neocortex as well as our primitive brain. It involves the whole human being. Homo sapiens will at last deserve that *"sapiens"* on the day when he puts his neocortical supercomputer at the service of life, at the service of a powerful attachment to life.

Notice, then, that the priorities suggested by our reflection on the genesis of an ecological Man are quite contrary to the priorities commonly proposed. For followers of intellectuals like Arthur Koestler, it is good form to refer to the insufficient domination of the neocortex over the irrational and extravagant archaic brain. Koestler was the author of books like *Janus* and *The Ghost in the Machine,* whose titles were in themselves significant. He dreamed discovering a combination of good enzymes that would give the neocortex the right of veto over the animal brain and thus correct a palpable error of evolution. This kind of absolute confidence in the intellect, plus apparent contempt for the wisdom of the instinctive brain — the brain that pushes to survive — can only lead to individual and collective suicide. The struggle for life is not rational. Let us recall that Koestler committed suicide. Let us take the opposite view from suicidal intellectuals. The point now is to rehabilitate the primitive brain, to put trust in its life-affirming powers when it has not been tamed during the period of dependency on the mother. The subduing of the primitive brain does not start with early and authoritarian potty-training — the education of our sphincters. It starts long before, as early as the first sucking.

Notes

1. In the realms of childbirth, other difficulties are specifically human, as well. Among other apes, the baby's head is smaller than the mother's pelvis, the mother's vulva is centered, and the baby's head does not have to describe a complex spiral to get out.

2. Modern nutritionists have recently developed the concept that certain fatty acids are essential to the brain. These are the "long-chain omega-3 polyunsaturated fatty acids," and are specific to the food chain of life in the sea.

CHAPTER EIGHT

Colostrum and Civilization

Colostrum is what the newborn baby finds in his mother's breast before the milk itself is available. It evokes the first sucking and is the symbol of instinct. But colostrum can also be regarded as a symbol of the repression of instinctive forces insofar as the baby of the cultural Man is usually deprived of it.

If you want to be struck with amazement by the matchless complexity of the physiological processes surrounding birth, if you want to discover their subtle intricacies, then spend a few hours, days, or months studying colostrum. Even then, you will have only scratched the surface of this huge topic, which can be approached in a number of ways.

First of all, let us look at what makes the colostrum produced in those very first hours so very special. It is a real concentration of antibodies, containing huge amounts of those substances that protect us against invaders, be they microbes, viruses, or another person's living cells. The most copious antibodies, called "IgA," cannot be made by the newborn itself and are not brought via the placenta. They are available during the first hours following birth in tens of milligrams per milliliter, and they protect the fragile mucous membranes of the bowels and of the respiratory tract. Their favorite targets are the microbes and viruses with which we have to cohabit from birth, since they are satellites of our mother.

In the colostrum of the first hours there are also millions of immune-active cells per cubic millimeter; the following week they can be counted only in the thousands. These macrophages and other kinds of white cells can neutralize and digest the most dangerous of germs. Colostrum is, in fact, an army able to suppress any kind of infection. It contains up to ten grams per liter of an ingenious anti-infection weapon called "lactoferrin." One molecule of lactoferrin can trap and smother two atoms of iron and thus starve and weaken bacteria, making them more vulnerable. Here we can draw up only a provisory list of these well-documented anti-infection agents, each working in its own way. Lysozym, interferon, the complement, and the ligands of folic acid are just some we could mention.

One has to understand that to be born is to enter the world of microbes. There are no microbes in the intestine of the fetus before birth; but within twenty-four hours afterward, there are billions of them per gram. If the baby has not been feeding, or has been given sugar and water or a "small" bottle of artificial milk, the microbes in his or her system will be quite different from those that will be present if he or she has taken only colostrum. The future of the intestinal flora depends on the first germs that occupy the territory. If the newborn baby has only consumed colostrum, the dominant microbes belong to the bifidobacterium family and are accompanied by some coliform bacteria to which the baby is already adapted, since they come from the mother. The newborn needs to be contaminated as early as possible by the domestic microbes that are satellites of its mother, and in this way be as well protected as possible in the event of an attack by more dangerous microbes.

In fact, it is unrealistic to dissociate the study of anti-infection strategies from the study of factors that reinforce the intestinal mucous membranes. At birth the intestine is very permeable to foreign proteins, viruses, microbial toxins, and germs. But the mucous membrane will get stronger all the more quickly the more colostrum the baby consumes. Growth factors such as taurine, and epidermal growth factors, speed up its proliferation. Other growth factors such as zinc have no special target, but are just as essential. It would be worth studying all the families of nutrients to learn what happens to them when colostrum becomes milk.

However, for the moment we will focus on the enormous quantity of fatty acids in colostrum — especially its long-chain polyunsaturated fatty acids, which are similar to those found in fish oils and in some precious plant oils such as evening primrose. This is an important topic because the human being is characterized by the huge development of the brain, and the brain is to a great extent made up of fatty substances. It is as if human colostrum was destined to meet the first nutritional needs of a big-brained ape adapted to the sea.

To study the inimitable complexity of colostrum is also to study the rapid changes in its concentrations of different nutrients and anti-infection substances.

Another amazing thing is the newborn baby's ability to search for the nipple, and to find it often as early as the first hour after birth. When mother and baby are comfortable in a warm place, in semidarkness, in close skin-to-skin contact with complete privacy, the baby finds the nipple soon indeed. What guides the baby toward the nipple? There are probably several factors at work, such as the small difference in temperature (about 0.5°C) between the nipple and the skin around it, and also the nipple's special odor. For this reason, it is important to avoid aggressive or overwhelming smells in a birth place.

Not only does the baby know how to find the breast; the mother also instinctively knows how to coordinate her own behavior with the newborn's while she is still under the influence of the hormones that made the delivery possible, and still in that special state of consciousness that tends to make her feel remote from our everyday world. This is what was going on at those times when I have seen women giving the breast half an hour after the birth although they had not planned to breastfeed.

I cannot help thinking of such scenes when intellectuals claim that human beings have no instinct. These people have never seen a mother and her newborn in an atmosphere of complete privacy, complete spontaneity. In the same way, the phrase *putting the baby to the breast* — often used to describe the first sucking — expresses a failure to recognize our instinctive potential in such circumstances. Speaking from my own experiences of home births, I can tell you that the baby invariably suckles during the first hour after birth — but nobody "puts the baby to the breast." Mother and baby coordinate their actions. The important thing is not to get in their way.

When experience and study have left you full of admiration for the properties of colostrum, and aware of the instinctive potential of human beings, you find yourself being tempted to ask the most seemingly innocent questions. This one, for instance: Are there societies so cruel that they would prevent or delay the consumption of this precious substance?

The answer to this question is a key to understanding the human phenomenon. In fact, most civilizations studied by historians and anthropologists have devised schemes to prohibit or to reduce the consumption of colostrum. And furthermore, some cultures consider colostrum to be tainted or harmful — even a substance to be expressed and discarded. This negative attitude toward colostrum is almost universal.

In many traditional African cultures, colostrum was likened to pus, or poison, and was therefore avoided. There have been precise reports to this effect in countries such as

Sierra Leone, Lesotho, and Malawi. Some tribes employ a specific ritual to ensure that the absorption of colostrum is hampered or postponed. For example, in the Bemba tribe in Zambia, the people put a small amount of gruel into the baby's mouth. They say it is to open up the mouth. Thereafter the mother can give the breast. Actually, the great behavioral maturity of the black African newborn babies compared with their white counterparts has passed more or less unnoticed up to now because the first contact between mother and baby is traditionally disturbed on the African continent. Recently a medical team in Malawi went against their own cultural beliefs and wondered whether early sucking might reduce the risks of hemorrhage after birth. In order to find out, they first of all had to experience and learn what happens when the period around birth is not disturbed at all. They could find no answers by reading a textbook. At the central hospital in Lilongwe, they tried to evaluate the average time from birth to the first sucking under undisturbed conditions. Since they had found no references to this in the national medical records, and thus had no preconceptions, they were not at all surprised to find that the mean time was around seven to eight minutes, with the fastest time being 3.5 minutes and the slowest, fifteen minutes. From my own experience I have found that, for a white baby, it is around three-quarters of an hour! And a Swedish midwife found it to be exactly fifty-five minutes!

There has always been a consensus of opinion in Asia that colostrum is bad. As far back as the second century B.C., Indian Ayurvedic medicine recommended honey and clarified butter for the newborn, while the colostrum was to be expressed and discarded. In Afghanistan the colostrum (called *fela*) was replaced by bitter herbs, sweets, and hyssop seeds. In Japan the elixir *Jumi Gokoto* was given to the newborn. This was made from nuts and herbs, but the specific ingredients were determined by caste; the highborns had more ingredients than the infants of the poor.

These attitudes and beliefs are deeply rooted, and thus they show up even in contemporary dress. In modern Korea, where 60–70 percent of babies are breastfed, breastfeeding does not start until the fourth day, the baby having been given formula for the first three days. Neither the doctors nor the mothers question this practice, which has to do with the separation of mother and baby while they are in hospital. It is significant that women accept this early separation without protest although no Korean mother would dream of leaving an older child's side in the hospital unless another family member took her place.

In China the routine is basically the same, with some local and regional variations. There also, the legacy of the past is reenacted. In every birthing place I visited in China in 1977, newborn babies up to the age of three days were refused the breast. Nothing has changed since that time, and now the Chinese are spending more time and energy mastering the technique of in-vitro fertilization than in studying and making known the properties of colostrum.

Negative attitudes toward colostrum are not uncommon in the American hemisphere either, and this has been noted particularly among the Indians of Guatemala. The Sioux, also, used to disturb the beginnings of the mother-newborn relationship quite openly; the consumption of colostrum was incompatible with their rituals. And, in the Yucatan peninsula, Brigitte Jordan studied the practice of a midwife who had preserved some of the ancestral traditions. These descendants of the Maya did not claim that colostrum was bad or that early sucking should be forbidden, but when one watches Brigitte's videotapes or reads her book or listens to her speaking about her Yucatan experiences, one becomes convinced that the early consumption of colostrum is made extremely difficult. Before the baby is in its mother's arms, the midwife gives it a routine bath, and then swaddles it; someone else may give it a little water to drink from a gourd dipper. And if the baby is a girl, she will even have her ears pierced before she is an hour old.

From stories told about births among the aborigines of Australia, we can conclude that the baby there could not find the breast immediately, either. Annette Hamilton, for example, studied childbirth in Arnhem Land, a part of the country that was virtually untouched by white development until 1930. It appears that the baby was first placed unwrapped into a bark cradle or directly onto a blanket, and then taken away by the woman's mother or sisters. In New Zealand, interestingly enough, the Maoris prove to be different from other oceanic cultures insofar as they do not hinder immediate sucking.

Western societies have always despised colostrum. In the sixth century B.C., Prokopios reported the customs of nomadic people in the northern parts of Sweden. There the newborn was immediately hung up in the trees, wrapped in fur skins, and given bone marrow to eat. In biblical times, colostrum was expressed and the baby given honey to cleanse the intestine before the proper milk was available. Greek doctors, Roman doctors, and then Western European doctors have shared the same beliefs. In the second century A.D., Soranus taught that mothers should wait for three weeks before giving the breast. In the Middle Ages, rosewater was commonly used as a purgative. Sometimes the mother was given an older child who was considered capable of digesting colostrum. In Brittany the baby was not put to the breast before baptism, at the age of two or three days. The Bretons of old believed that, if the baby swallowed milk before the ceremony, the devil might enter the baby's body with the milk.

In Tudor and Stuart England, colostrum was openly regarded as a harmful substance, to be discarded. The mother was not considered to be "clean" after childbirth until the bloody discharge called "lochia" had stopped flowing. She was not permitted to give the breast until after a religious service of purification and thanksgiving called "churching." Meanwhile the baby was given various types of purgative such as butter and honey and sugar or oil of sweet almonds, or sugared wine. Paintings from that time show the new-born infant fed with a spoon while the mother recovers in bed.

The first Western doctor who dissented from his colleagues by praising colostrum and advocating breastfeeding from birth onward was probably William Cadogan, at the end of the eighteenth century. In fact his ulterior motive was to purge the baby, but he had observed that colostrum is also a purgative. It is probably not coincidental that the infant mortality rate dropped dramatically in Great Britain around that time. But Cadogan's influence did not last long, and few Western babies were allowed colostrum during the nineteenth and twentieth centuries. In the 1970s when I described the sort of atmosphere that facilitates the first sucking, many people at the conference thought I was spinning a yarn.

Today, only twenty years later, nobody would openly question the irreplaceable value of colostrum. It is currently fashionable to state that the baby should be "put to the breast" as soon as possible. But, in fact, it is still a disturbing topic, and "serious people" have better things to do than to study it thoroughly.

Go to a medical or scientific library and look up colostrum in the catalog. It won't take more than a few minutes to realize that veterinary surgeons publish more on the subject than doctors for humans do. Of course, antibodies do not pass through the placenta of bovines as easily as through that of humans, but this is not the main reason. Breeders of race horses know that a foal deprived of colostrum will never be a champion.

I think that people try to appease any feelings of guilt they may have about this dismal state of human affairs, by praising colostrum every now and again. But actually the conditions prevailing around birth in our society mean that babies cannot consume it precociously and completely. First, in the context of a big modern hospital, very few women can achieve the complex hormonal balance that makes a normal birth possible. They need a variety of substitutes for their own hormones — substitutes that profoundly disturb the whole continuum of the physiological process. Then, as soon as the baby is born, there is always something more urgent to do than to protect the privacy of the mother and baby. They are often surrounded by an army of people bustling around. A synthetic hormone is injected into the mother to facilitate the detachment of the placenta. The attendants cannot wait to cut the cord. And even after it has emitted a powerful scream, the baby's throat is aspirated. No one feels any hesitation about looking at the perineum with a bright light. The Apgar score is assessed. Eye drops must be administered urgently. The baby must be weighed and checked for abnormalities. The placenta must be inspected. There must be no delay in washing the room and thinking about the next birth. The baby's first night is spent in a nursery because the mother needs a rest. There is no hesitation in giving the infant some sugar water or a little formula milk.

And there are many subtle and indirect ways, as well, to inhibit the contact between mother and her newborn. For example, as discussed in Chapter 4, it is now commonplace to encourage early direct father-baby bonding, at the risk of diminishing the role of the father as the protector of mother and baby as a unit.

When we start trying to match up the scientifically demonstrated beneficial quality of colostrum and the more or less universal rejection of it, we are naturally prompted to think that there is probably *some* reason for the rejection. And so we go in search of an explanation.

The anthropologist Margaret Mead is one of the very few

researchers who have raised this question and proposed an answer. She suggested that the lack of colostrum might have an effect on genetic selection. Only those babies who are the most suited to surviving the hazards of the perinatal period can do so in such a state of deprivation. This explanation is difficult to accept, however, because it is most unusual for the process of natural selection to unfold at the price of deliberately weakening the health of all the members of the group.

I propose another interpretation. Man emerged as a species several million years ago. Since then tribes have eliminated other tribes, civilizations have wiped out other civilizations, and human groups have gradually mastered the animal and plant kingdoms. The only human groups having descendants on the planet over the past few thousand years are those who knew how to cultivate the human capacity to destroy life most efficiently. They are those who had the best means of achieving this goal at their disposal. The most efficient way to make Man a superpredator is to disturb the mother-newborn relationship. Claiming that colostrum is bad is an easy way of weakening this relationship; and so, doing so has — up to now — been an advantage in terms of selection.

In fact, the deprivation of colostrum is just one example of the cultural Man's potential for cruelty toward the newborn baby, and for meddling in the baby's relationship with his or her mother. Neonatal circumcision, tight swaddling, baptism by immersion in cold water, "smoking" the baby, piercing the ears of little girls, opening the doors in cold countries, all have the same meaning. When Igor Tcharkovsky immerses a baby in icy water or subjects babies to various contortions with the intention of adapting them to water or making them strong or developing their spiritual strength, I find it difficult to accept this as the work of a pioneer; it is more like going back to the past.

This sort of behavior made sense at a time when every

human group was intent on dominating the others as well as other plant and animal species, and when humanity as a whole was bent on dominating the planet. In the current age of ecological consciousness, however, these priorities are obsolete, and even reversed. Today the priority is to stop destroying the biosphere and to maintain a positive attitude toward life. Cruelty toward the newborn baby no longer makes sense.

What's more, my interpretation is borne out when one considers those civilizations that have been able to survive without following the usual strategies. They isolated themselves in territory that nobody else wanted and that could not be reached easily by others. They integrated themselves effortlessly with the ecosystem. People like the Huichols in northwestern Mexico, the Pygmies in the deep equatorial forests, and the Maoris who settled in New Zealand, all lived in remote parts of the world and were protected by geography until the nineteenth century. The main feature that these cultures have in common is a deeply rooted sense of ecology, a kind of ecological instinct. The Huichols talk about "the other world" when they refer to the destructive madness of other humans. The Pygmies have an enormous respect for trees, and the Maoris worship Mother Earth. Another similarity is that the very beginning of the mother-baby relationship is not disturbed, and thus it seems that colostrum can be consumed unreservedly.

A comparative study of cultures inevitably leads us to compare the mother-baby relationship and the relationship of humanity with Mother Earth. Of course, some human groups have openly drawn this parallel. For example, the Sioux thought of the ideal man as courageous and an aggressive warrior. The ideal woman was the wife or sister of such a man. The Sioux would say quite plainly that in order to attain this warrior ideal they had to prevent any intimate contact between the newborn baby and its mother, and also prevent any immediate contact between the newborn and

the earth. For this reason, at the time of the birth, four courageous warriors would grab the corners of the blanket on
which the woman was lying, lift the blanket, and hold it up
a little distance from the ground. In their own way, they
knew about what modern scientists call "that sensitive
period" — that is to say, one of those developmentally important short periods of time that will never happen again.

The revolution we are waiting for will have a global di-
mension. We will call it "the colostral revolution." This revolution implies changes of attitude that will be radical in
the literal sense of the word because we will have to take
our deepest roots and our mammalian past into account.
Normally speaking, mammals — and in particular our cousins the primates — are not cruel to their newborn babies.
How did humans become what they are today? A recent experiment involving marmosets is significant in this regard.
In a natural environment the she-monkey leaves her group
during the night, perches in a treetop, and gives birth to her
twins. A scientist studying captive marmosets artificially
eliminated the night element of the day-night cycle and
kept the lights on constantly. The females were disturbed by
this situation and had long and difficult labors. Another interesting fact was the incredible nervousness and dangerous
need for activity among the other members of the group as
soon as a baby was born. Some would start eating the placenta and — probably by accident — a baby or two as well.

Such a story gives us an inkling of the reasons why female
mammals isolate themselves to give birth to their offspring.
It is not to hide from their predators, but to be protected
from the uncontrolled activity of the other members of the
group.

We begin to understand that many aggressive rituals,
passed on from generation to generation, are actually different variants of deeply rooted behavior. Many medical practices that doctors rationalize afterward can be interpreted in
this light. For example, the need to watch and to cut the

perineum is hard to justify now that controlled studies have been published that suggest the main risk factors in terms of serious tears are, in fact, episiotomy and having to lie on the back with the legs up in stirrups. Another example is the compulsion to cut the cord immediately although there is no overriding reason for suddenly interrupting the flow of blood between the baby and its placenta. It would be impossible to enumerate all the medical interventions that have been proposed and practiced in the period of excitation following a birth. Suction of the newborn baby's stomach is commonly practiced in some hospitals, despite the fact that the gastric juices contain a lot of important substances— such as the hormone gastrin, which plays a part in the movements of the digestive tract.

In some countries, such as the United States, circumcision soon after birth is a common practice, even without any religious motivation. Doctors justify their attitude in this by presenting comparative statistics on urinary infections. But if the prevention of infection were the main preoccupation, birth at home among familiar microbes would be encouraged, and under conditions that make the early and complete absorption of colostrum easy.

The denial of the need for privacy, which resulted in a depreciation of colostrum and the development of interruptive rituals and aggressive medical practices, is the primary phenomenon. It is the denial of our mammalian condition and should be the starting point for the colostral revolution, which really is therefore a matter of "counter Culture." The aim is to rediscover the real priorities and may countermand usual human behavior. These days it is considered good form to stress the need for help, support, and so to suggest that a woman cannot give birth by herself. The compulsion to help is sometimes difficult to dissociate from the need to observe and to control, and often conflicts with the need for privacy of the person supposedly being helped.

The colostral revolution *must* happen as part of the

process of harmonizing our instincts and our science as they derive from the primitive brain and the neocortex, respectively. This is not just a utopian theory, because in fact the process has already begun.

It is worth pointing out some significant symptoms of this truly countercultural phenomenon. The first baby son of a Jewish woman was born in a conventional hospital and was circumcised according to tradition. The second baby boy was born at home in complete privacy, on the floor, close to the bed, without any medical interference. He found the breast immediately and started suckling vigorously without any delay. Nobody separated him from his mother, so they maintained skin-to-skin contact day and night. In spite of family pressure, the child was not circumcised. His mother had retained her capacity to protect her newborn baby intact, and her maternal instinct held 4,000-year-old doctrines in check.

This example is not unique. The colostral revolution will bring about a reconsideration of many received ideas regarding the newborn baby. For example, it has always been considered normal for the newborn baby to lose weight during the first two or three days, and to recover his birth weight at about eight days old. This is supposedly "physiological" weight loss. It was already a well-accepted phenomenon at the beginning of this century when most babies were born at home. And neonatal weight loss is still taken for granted in modern textbooks written by experts whose only experience of birth is in obstetric departments. It is regarded simply as a matter of fact and is not usually discussed or reconsidered, even in those birthing centers where they try not to disturb the beginning of the mother-baby relationship or the beginning of breastfeeding and where the baby can find the breast immediately as well as share the mother's bed.

Home birth gave me the opportunity to observe new kinds of babies — babies who have already spent two hours suckling vigorously at the age of three hours; babies who are kept in skin-to-skin contact with their mothers day and night, in a familiar place. Among them, one baby out of three does not lose weight at all and is heavier than its birth weight at the age of a week. From these babies, we learn that weight loss is not mandatory. Perhaps it is not physiological either, even if it has been the rule in most human cultures.

Up till now the physiologists have interpreted the phenomenon they were observing as being the consequence of a water loss necessary in adapting to life in the atmosphere. Now we must explain how it is that some babies do not lose weight at all. The main reason is probably that we have always underestimated the amount of colostrum a baby can consume within the first couple of hours, especially after a fetus ejection reflex. The colostrum of the first hours has an enormous concentration of antibodies — proteins having huge osmotic pressure, that is to say, a huge capacity to retain water. It also contains a variety of nutrients and growth factors that stimulate the main metabolic pathways. Besides, we can safely assume that a newborn baby who has been welcomed into the arms of an ecstatic mother, and covered with a warm blanket in a warm place, is in a hormonal balance that involves a minimal loss of energy.

Premature and low-birth-weight babies should be the first to benefit from the colostral revolution. In the days when there were no incubators, babies weighing only one kilogram (or about 2.2 pounds) survived. There have been famous cases of this kind. The attendants used to wrap such a baby in cotton and lay her or him close to the fire or in a bed of feathers. Apparently, it never occurred to them to consider the warmth of the mother's body, the pleasure of skin-to-skin contact, or the qualities of colostrum. What I have learned with full-term babies born at home applies to most premature babies as well. Indeed, it is especially important for them to be born as easily as possible without any drugs, among domestic germs, and held directly against the mother's skin, day and night, like baby kangaroos. Up to now, though, I have never been called to a premature birth at home. Given the current medical context of birthing, the rate of prematurity is very low among women whose choice is to give birth at home.

The "kangaroo method" was initially conceived as a way to reconsider the pros and cons of the incubator. An incubator is nothing more than a cage made of glass and a thermostat. Its only function is to provide warmth. But a baby in an incubator is deprived of skin stimulation. Hence, the so-called TLCs (tender loving carers) were invented in the United States. This means that a zealous nurse stimulates the baby's skin according to a pre-established protocol. Moreover, a baby in an incubator is not mobilized, and thus the inner ear (the vestibular system) lacks essential stimulation. Hence, the oscillating bed was invented. Furthermore, the baby cannot perceive significant sounds. Hence, recordings of the mother's voice were piped into the incubator at one Paris hospital. (But soon it was discovered that the sound of waves had the same effect on the baby and, in the long run, was more tolerable for the nursing team.) Finally, it has also been demonstrated that the sense of smell has a role to play in identifying the mother. Hence, a piece of linen impregnated with the mother's odor was introduced into the incubator.

If we add that the germs found in an incubator are quite unlike the germs that are satellites of the mother, and that the mother who is separated from her baby is not in the best condition to secrete milk, one wonders why nobody thought of the kangaroo method earlier. Why did it not occur to anyone that the mother might be the best possible incubator? The baby is placed in a pouch and held close to the breast, in contact with its mother's skin day and night, in an upright position in a very warm room.

The phrase *kangaroo baby* used in reference to premature

babies comes from Bogota, Colombia. Actually, when I went there in 1981 I did not hear this expression, but they had already reconsidered the conventional approach, as a result of lack of incubators, lack of well-trained nurses, and a huge number of premature babies. The new policy made it possible for all the premature babies — whatever their weight — to stay in touch with their mother's body and go home, provided they were breathing autonomously. The rate of survival increased dramatically, particularly in babies lighter than a kilogram.

We were already thinking along the same lines in Pithiviers. Between 1978 and 1984, there were 100 premature babies born at our maternity hospital who were kept with their mothers day and night like real kangaroos, rather than being transferred to a specialized center. We found advantages in this: not having to interrupt the skin-to-skin contact in the first minutes after birth, and avoiding the inconvenience of a transferral from one hospital unit to another.

One might suppose that such an attitude would spread quickly all over the world — but not so. In the wealthy countries, it is commonly claimed that such a simple method would only be good for the Third World. And in most Third World countries, birthing policies are deeply influenced by the traditional beliefs about colostrum as well as by the desire to be seen as modern. However, the kangaroo baby cannot be dissociated from the big colostral revolution that is underway in many various and separate places.

The babies of the colostral age will be very different from those the experts know at the present time. Most neonatal experts and pediatricians forget to warn us that they only know about one kind of baby: the baby born in the hospital, who does not sleep with his or her mother and who is weaned before the age of one. I feel more and more familiar with a new sort of human baby, unknown by most experts. One of the objects of our recently created Primal Health Research Center in London will be to observe such babies throughout their lives. But some obvious differences can be detected even as early as the first few days of life, without sophisticated statistics. For example, babies who start suckling during the hour following birth are very seldom jaundiced, or their jaundice is quite mild, particularly if they were born at home and sleep with their mother. This might be easily explained by the fact that these babies did not share a glucose IV drip with their mothers during birth and that, generally speaking, they have not received any drugs. Drugs are well-known factors influencing the severity of neonatal jaundice. But the main factor involved is probably the colostrum itself, and the action of suckling, which stimulates the movement of the intestinal tract so that the bilirubin pigment cannot be reabsorbed in any great quantity and thus return to the bloodstream.

While the consumption of colostrum and the birthing context that makes it possible have visible and even measurable short-term effects, the colostral revolution is associated with the hope of long-term effects, and primarily on the health of the individual. Is life expectancy longer when colostrum has been consumed? Are you likely to get ulcerative colitis if you had colostrum at the beginning of your life? Thousands of questions like these have never been asked, and that is the reason why the Primal Health Research Center was founded.

Profound effects on our mental outlook are also expected. The exceptional societies that survived into historic times in spite of their respect for colostrum had no aggression toward Mother Earth. On the contrary, they venerated her. The colostral revolution is thus also the fusion of the image of the Mother and the image of Mother Earth.

It is literally a revolution because it implies coming full circle and returning to our mammalian nature even while heralding a new departure. It is not sufficient just to teach that colostrum contains antibodies and that the baby should be put to the breast as soon as possible. We are speaking here of much more than a method that might be introduced without changing the whole context.

It will be difficult for some people to understand the real nature of this revolution — probably as difficult as it has been for some people to understand the direction we took in Pithiviers in the early 1970s. There are those for whom Pithiviers was the maternity hospital where pregnant women sang; for some, it was the homelike birthing rooms; for others, the pool, or giving birth in an upright position, or in the dark. For still others, it was the role given to the midwives, or the kangaroo babies, or a perinatal mortality rate below 10 per 1,000 as early as 1976.

Each of these images of Pithiviers, taken out of context, tends to hide the reality. Pithiviers was much more than the sum of its parts.

CHAPTER NINE

From Holland to Malawi

Having given a cross-cultural consideration to colostrum and civilization, let us now go back to Holland and Malawi, focusing on these two countries to which we have referred already.

A list of the main reports that ring the death knell of the electronic age in birthing is an essential document for anyone wishing to understand the radical changes to which we are participating.[1] In the same way, we cannot prepare for the post-electronic age without examining closely a number of amazing statistics from Holland.

In 1985, there were 179,190 babies born in the Netherlands. In the same year the Dutch perinatal mortality rate (that is, the number of babies who died after six months in the womb and before the age of one week) was 9.8 per thousand, and the rate of cesarean section was around 6 percent. No other nation in the world has ever achieved such a low perinatal mortality rate associated with such a low rate of cesareans. Countries where the perinatal mortality rate is now even lower than the rate in Holland in 1985 are those that are using routine ultrasound scans during the second trimester of pregnancy; in this way, they replace some perinatal deaths with some abortions for gross abnormalities. Incidentally, our figures in Pithiviers (without the use of scans) were roughly the same as the Dutch — but that was on the scale of a hospital, rather than a state!

So what is the Dutch secret? Why is Holland so special?

In the same year, 65,518 Dutch babies were born at home — that is to say, 36.6 percent of the total. These figures make Holland an exception in the developed world. In all the other developed countries, the rate of home birth is below 2 percent, and often close to 0 percent. Let us add that, while the overall perinatal mortality rate in Holland was 9.8 per thousand (which is itself excellent), the mortality rate for the babies born at home was only 1.9 per thousand.

Some local Dutch statistics provide further details and give us still more food for thought. For example, a study made in Wormerveer, a suburb of Amsterdam, showed that, between 1969 and 1983, there were 7,980 women booked originally at the midwives' practice. As it turned out, 74.9 percent of them gave birth with their midwife as they had planned, either at home or in a small birthing center. In this group, the perinatal mortality rate was 1.3 per thousand. Another 8 percent were referred to an obstetrician during labor or delivery; and in this group, the perinatal mortality rate was 11 per thousand (better than the overall Dutch rate in the same period). The rest — 17.1 percent — were referred to an obstetrician during pregnancy with the label *high-risk;* and in this group, the perinatal mortality rate was 51.7 per thousand.

There are several complementary interpretations of this fascinating data. The first is that the midwives — who are responsible for the selection procedure during pregnancy — are very shrewd. The strong point of the system is that the right people are doing the screening: those who have enormous experience of what is normal, so that they can detect very quickly any cause for concern. They probably not only take heed of official criteria, but also take into account their own intuitions. In the hospital at Pithiviers, some of the help nurses had changed diapers for thousands and thousands of newborn babies by the end of their careers. Very often they were the ones who detected — usually in a matter of seconds — anything unusual or worrisome.

Another interpretation of the Dutch figures is that the label *high risk* is, itself, dangerous in terms of the anxiety it triggers and maintains over a period of several months.

From my own experience of home birth I have come to the conclusion that, in most cases, the first stage of labor — that is, the period of dilation — is the best time to detect the women who should not give birth at home. The first stage of labor is the only time when the quality of the uterine contractions can be evaluated by an experienced birth attendant. As a general rule, the risks are minimal when the first stage has been straightforward. (Of course, an evaluation of the physiological potential of the laboring woman is only possible in an atmosphere of complete privacy.) Thus, following this strategy, I do not refuse to attend a woman for a home birth in advance of the onset of labor just because she happens to be expecting her first baby at age forty, or expecting her first baby who is in a breech position, or because she has had a previous cesarean section, for example. It is not too late to make a decision about the ultimate place of birth during the first stage of labor.

I wonder if, in some cases, the Dutch midwives would not be better off postponing as much as possible their decision to transfer to an obstetrician. As it happens, they have very good outcomes after transferring during labor.

We also have a lot to learn from some amazing statistics coming from the Third World. As mentioned in Chapter 8, a medical team in Malawi — whose members wanted to study the risks of hemorrhage after birth — developed an educational program for the traditional midwives. During refresher courses, some groups of midwives were trained to go beyond their cultural beliefs and to put the baby to the breast as soon as possible after birth. They were told that the reasons for this practice are that it helps to keep the baby warm, that it results in earlier successful lactation as well as prolonged breastfeeding, and that it promotes bonding. Other groups of midwives were not taught this practice and were supposed to be the control group. In fact, no clear conclusion could be drawn about the blood loss insofar as the researchers were comparing a practice that was against cultural beliefs with a traditional practice.

But thanks to this study, one of the most comprehensive investigations ever recorded about the practice of traditional birth attendants came to be published. These traditional midwives have impressive results, considering that they live and practice in conditions such that the nearest telephone or health center is often more than three miles away. When the suckling and the control groups are looked at together, one finds that, over a period of about six months, sixty-nine midwives attended 4,227 deliveries. In this series there was only one maternal death (after transfer to a hospital), there were thirty-five stillbirths (0.8%), and four babies died before the age of one week (0.1%). Let us add that there were twenty-seven perineal tears, no episiotomies, and four transfers for retained placenta. There were eighteen twin babies in this series, all of them born alive.

Of course, it is possible to claim that there was some pre-labor screening and that the average number of babies per woman in Malawi is higher than in a developed country. Nonetheless, these figures are essential data for all those concerned with the ecology of birth. They would be acceptable even in a wealthy country with surgical facilities, blood transfusions, and high-tech resuscitation on hand for everyone.

These statistics from Holland and Malawi suggest that the attitude toward childbirth held by the society as a whole is probably more important than any strategic details that might be taught during workshops. They also confirm the importance of being deeply integrated within one's human community. Perhaps one reason why giving birth is often difficult in a country like the United States is that very few people have strong links with their human environment. Once, at the end of a workshop in Hawaii, I asked the participants how many of them were still living in the city where they were born. Not one hand was raised. It is difficult to go back to your roots when your roots are distant and weak. It is also difficult to go back to your roots when your daily language as an adult is not your mother tongue. Nowadays this is a common situation.

People who are deeply integrated into their community, such as those who have spent their whole life in a traditional small village, are constantly overcontrolled and observed. They are never anonymous. They are not vulnerable to a lack of privacy. In some cultures, women can even give birth in a passageway or a bush-covered shelter in full view of everyone, including their own children. This is the case of the Jarara in South America, as reported by Niles Newton. Modern women, on the other hand, often have an anonymous life in a big city and can easily become isolated in their own bathrooms. On the day when they give birth, they are extremely vulnerable to a lack of privacy.

The statistics from Holland and Malawi also confirm the importance of experienced birth attendants. A highly educated Dutch midwife and an illiterate and innumerate Malawi traditional birth attendant have their tremendous experience of birth in common. The greater your experience of birth, the less contagious fear you transmit. In terms of contagious fear, how would we even start to compare a Malawi-type of birth and a modern "husband-coached" delivery?!

Note

1. See the references listed under "Chapter 2" in the Selected Bibliography.

CHAPTER TEN

Photos and Videos

The epidemic is well established. The time has come to re-press it. The epidemic of photos and videos, I mean. We ourselves have indeed played a great part in the spread of this epidemic. There was a time when it was imperative to do away with many of the old mental images associated with words like *delivery* and *birth*. The point — and we felt it to be urgent — was to put forward pictures that showed alternatives to childbirth with the mother on a table, under bright lights, surrounded by guides and coaches.

Now, the priority is to rediscover the need for privacy, and the importance of dim lights. We must learn to eliminate *all* the onlookers and all their different ways of observing.

When participating in TV programs or reports with photographs, we were certainly aware of the need for privacy. That is why we were always anxious to introduce the camera only at the very last moment, just before the birth, at the point of no return when there is no risk of stopping the progress of the delivery. We always avoided making pictures during the first stage of labor, and we were very cautious before the delivery of the placenta. I remember one woman who delivered her baby right in front of a big German TV camera and said some minutes afterward, "It was wonderful! What a pity there was nobody to take a picture!"

This period is over. Films and photos cannot demonstrate the need for privacy and the importance of darkness. A camera is even more invasive at home than in a hospital. That is why, in this book, there are no photos of birth. The post-electronic age, the colostral age, is also the post-photographic age.

CHAPTER ELEVEN

Freud as a Midwife

The goats have no midwives. The sheep have no mid-
wives.
   When the goat is pregnant she is safely delivered.
   When the sheep is pregnant she is safely delivered.
You, in this state of pregnancy, will be safely delivered.
                              —Recited by the village midwife and several
                                  elders among the African Yoruba

We usually think of a midwife as a woman who attends
women in labor, encouraging, supporting, even coaching
them, and communicating by talking or touching. It is less
usual to refer to another kind of midwife — one who keeps a
low profile and just sits unseen in a corner or even in an adjoining room. But in fact, this low-profile midwifery probably creates the best possible situation in which to facilitate
the change of consciousness that is specific to the normal
process of birth.

Only a laboring woman who does not feel observed can
easily "surrender," and "go to another planet." Let us translate this concept into modern scientific language and say
that in such a situation it is easier to reduce neocortical con-

trol, and that a reduction of neocortical control is a prerequisite for a normal, physiologically directed delivery.

I cannot help recalling the breakthrough Freud made in
our understanding of human nature when he started to sit
unseen in a corner and when he discarded authoritarian
hypnosis. "Free association" became possible. Saying whatever comes to mind became a basic tool in exploring the unconscious. Psychoanalysis was born. We will never know for
sure which factor was really influential in originating this
radical change of attitude. Perhaps Freud took serious account of the story of Anna, who dared to ask her therapist
Joseph Breuer — a friend of Freud — to let her talk and
"chimney sweep." Who knows? Or perhaps Freud wanted to
avoid sexual provocation by female patients under hypnosis.
It is also possible that, originally, Freud wanted primarily to
protect his own privacy and not to become too personally
involved.

The important point is that he opened a new phase in the
understanding of human nature just by staying in the background and keeping a low profile. We at the end of this century refer often to Freudian theories but tend to forget how
extraordinary, how revolutionary, was the method he introduced. New interpretations can be proposed today for
things Freud could not explain easily in the scientific context of the end of the nineteenth century. One can now understand that a certain reduction in neocorticol control is a
prerequisite to exploring the unconscious, and that privacy
is a factor facilitating a reduction of neocorticol control.

The concept of privacy should be associated with the advent of psychoanalysis. Why is this not so? The first reason
might be that most Western languages do not have an
equivalent word for *privacy* at their disposal. They cannot
use one precise and useful word that simply means the state
of not feeling observed, with a positive connotation. In
French, Italian, and Spanish, the nearest words are *in-*

timité, intimità, and *intimidad,* respectively, which are
the equivalent of the English *intimacy.* The translator of
one of my books in German associated the concepts of
privatsphare and *intimsphare* to try to cover the whole content of the word *privacy.* I remember interpreters in Athens
arguing violently about the best translation in modern
Greek.

Why are so many languages deprived of a concept that
corresponds to this deeply rooted need in all mammals to
isolate themselves to give birth and to die? The answer is
probably that most known human cultures have denied the
mammalian need for privacy at birth and at death for such
a long time that the very concept has been lost, and hence
so has the relevant word.

These considerations are not purely academic. They are
of paramount importance now, at the end of the electronic
age in childbirth, at a time when it would be beneficial in
many countries to increase significantly the ratio of midwives to obstetricians. It is clear that the birth outcomes are
much better in countries—like Sweden, Holland, and the
United Kingdom—where midwives dramatically outnum-
ber obstetricians and where midwifery is a well-established
profession, compared with countries—like the United
States, Canada, Brazil, and Italy—where there are fewer
midwives or where they are looked on as mere auxiliaries of
the doctors.

Not only must the number of midwives versus obstetricians be reconsidered, but we have also to redefine authentic midwifery. Today the same word has different meanings.
There are huge differences between a European midwife
who has been trained for several years in the obstetric de-
partment of a teaching hospital and has never seen a birth
outside this context, and a home-birth midwife in Texas
who learned her skills via apprenticeship. In the United
States, the same word is used to designate one who is prac-

ticing "spiritual midwifery" at the Farm, in Columbia, Tennessee, for example, and a so-called certified nurse midwife who is a member of a hospital medical team.

One cannot redefine authentic midwifery without recalling the different phases through which midwifery has passed in the history of mankind, and even in the history of the mammals. The roots of midwifery can be found in the behavior of certain mammals. At the birth of a baby elephant, there is often an experienced female present, and other females gather to make a protective outward-looking circle around the mother. At the birth of a baby dolphin, there is also often a female present who can help the newborn to reach the surface and take its first breath. The other members of the group mount guard and are ready to kill any marauding sharks. It seems that among the mammals, when there is a "midwife," she is first of all a protector.

Among humans, the original midwife was probably the mother of the birth-giver or a substitute for the mother — an experienced close relative such as an aunt or a grandmother. At this stage of history, women were probably still isolating themselves by a river or a spring, or in a bush, or in a special hut or some other small dark place. One can imagine that the mother-midwife was behaving like a mother looking after her child in a playground. The child tends to forget her presence so long as everything is going well. It is not by chance that in many languages the root of the word meaning *midwife* is a word that means *mother* (*matrone, matrona*). The mother-midwife is primarily a protector; she is somebody you can call urgently, and who is immediately available in case of unexpected difficulties.

At a later stage in the history of humanity, a certain degree of specialization entered society. The midwife was chosen from among the most experienced women of the community. Her wisdom and her charisma were then expected to be her main qualities. She tends gradually to help, rather than to protect. She is supposed to have power, like a shaman. This could be the power to be in touch with the spirits via specific prayers or to use efficacious herbs, or to practice a traditional technique of massage. It is through her that the community can interfere in the process of birth. This led to the age of professionalism, and women did not give birth anymore; they were delivered by an experienced person. At the end of this long and complicated process, the word *midwife* is still used to refer to a technician, male or female, an anonymous member of a medical team. Nancy Cohen calls some of these modern midwives FLAMES — Female Labor Assistants who are Medically or Establishment Supportive. In this context, the mother-to-be is a patient.

What kind of midwife shall be needed in the future? The usual answer nowadays is to say that we need a woman who will afford emotional support (especially in America), or who will provide "care" (especially in England). The tendency is always to reconfirm the deeply imprinted belief that nobody can give birth without some kind of mysterious energy coming from outside. It is unusual to insist on the need for privacy and its corollary, the need for protection. It is unusual to go back to the roots of midwifery. However, this is probably just what we need — not least, in order to understand better the physiological processes of birth.

The low-profile midwife able to sit unseen in a corner has a knowledge of the process of birth that is not shared by the type of midwife who needs first and foremost to be actively supporting and helping. Just as Freud triggered a breakthrough in our interpretation of human behavior by staying in the background, in the same way a midwife who does not work obtrusively, and does not guide, can radically change our understanding of the birth process. Thanks to his approach, Freud discovered so-called transference, the process by which an individual's feelings shift from one person to another. A parallel can be made with the role that some authentic midwives feel is theirs: when they just keep a low profile, stay in the background, they feel they are a substitute for the mother. Thus, they see themselves as the object of a transference; they have heard hundreds of women calling for their mommas while in hard labor.

The fact that some laboring women seem to communicate with their own mothers, if only through a substitute, highlights the great importance of the work done by John Kennell and Marshall Klaus on the subject of the *doula*. A doula is a mother who has had no nursing or medical training but who has personally experienced normal vaginal births with good outcomes. She stays continuously with the laboring woman. Kennell and Klaus started their studies in the 1970s in two busy hospitals in Guatemala where fifty to sixty babies are born every day and where the routines have been established by doctors and nurses from the United States. They found that the presence of a doula reduces dramatically the incidence of all sorts of intervention and the use of drugs, and improves the outcome. Recently the researchers reproduced their study in Houston, Texas, in a neighborhood where the population is predominantly Hispanic and incomes are low. The birthing care-givers there are directed by English-speaking residents in a twelve-bed ward. The doulas speak both Spanish and English. As in Guatemala, the presence of a doula has obvious positive effects here, too. My own interpretation is that, in such an unfamiliar and strange environment, the doula is felt to be a protector. She is as protective as a mother would be.

The doula can also be seen as link with daily life insofar as she looks like, speaks like, and behaves like any other woman belonging to the community. This makes me think of the advice given to the women who give birth at the Garden Hospital in London: "Bring some familiar objects with you from home." It is difficult to have a feeling of privacy in a completely unfamiliar environment. Of course, Kennell and Klaus interpret their results according to the dominant beliefs of our time. They use the word *support* rather than the words *privacy* and *protection.*

Whatever interpretations are drawn from them, these studies should contribute to a radical change in the current birthing practices of the industrialized countries. They are contemporary and complement the many statistics tending to demonstrate that electronic fetal monitoring does more harm than good. The way the doulas are chosen should be an inspiration in countries that are rediscovering midwifery, such as Canada and the United States, as well as in the European countries where midwifery is well established. In France, for instance, women (and men) who apply to enter a midwifery school are selected by means of theoretical written exams. It is altogether possible that if, instead of these exams, they began to use the criteria used to choose the doulas, the obstetric statistics might be improved. Of course, the criteria of selection to enter a midwifery program are never perfect, and I do know women who have had no babies of their own and who are, nevertheless, good midwives. The point is that a woman who has given birth normally is guaranteed to be the kind of person whose presence will not disturb a woman in labor, while a good knowledge of the structure of the mitochondria does not carry the same guarantee.

When discussing the optimum number of midwives versus obstetricians, and when considering how the candidates for midwifery training might be selected in the future, we are projecting ourselves into the twenty-first century. To emphasize the need for privacy is also to enter the field of long-term visions. The need for privacy — which does not mean loneliness — has been denied for so many thousands of years that it cannot be thoroughly understood overnight. It is not so difficult, for example, to criticize the delivery position that has been adopted for the past three centuries. And it is easy also to propose a birthing pool to facilitate the first stage of labor. The *really* countercultural and revolutionary proposals are the ones that stress the need for privacy. But in all our discussions, we have to keep in mind those who will be having babies in the transitional phase of the history of childbirth, and who will have to adapt to an environment that is still not best designed to avoid the use of drugs. Avoiding drugs might indeed become the main objective in the foreseeable future since we are becoming more and more aware of the probable long-term negative side effects of all the drugs used during labor, while it has been more difficult, so far, to demonstrate any long-term negative effects of the different mechanical ways used to assist birth — for example, forceps, suction, cesarean section.

One can assume that, during this period of transition, different substitutes for privacy might be helpful and easier to introduce than privacy itself. Self-hypnosis might be one of the techniques adapted to the present situation. Pregnant women trained to use this technique can "switch off completely" at will, and escape from reality. This is not basically any different from the techniques of visualization, or multisensory visualization, or guided imagery used in the United States in particular, or from the *sophrologie* used in the French- and Spanish-speaking countries.

The term *self-hypnosis* has the big advantage of stressing the capacity to maintain one's own autonomy. Self-hypnosis shares little in common with the authoritarian hypnosis that has been used in obstetrics for a long time and that implies a dependency on the hypnotist.

Having alluded to hypnosis, I should point out that the altered states of consciousness that accompany physiological processes such as labor and orgasm have not been studied as seriously as the states of consciousness artificially induced by hypnosis, different meditation techniques, drugs, and so forth. Nobody knows, for example, what an electroencephalogram[1] looks like during the different phases of labor or during an orgasm. Such paradoxical ignorance can be interpreted several ways. First, it reflects the current lack of interest in the physiological processes at work in the period surrounding birth, and the common reluctance to consider sexual life as a whole. Second, any such studies would face huge difficulties insofar as all the episodes of sexual life are highly dependent on the environment, and especially on the degree of privacy pertaining. In spite of the difficulties, though, I am convinced that one day there will be attempts made to learn from these kinds of exploration. It might provoke a new way of looking at sexuality as a whole if the change of consciousness experienced by the mother during a fetus ejection reflex turns out not to differ fundamentally from the change of consciousness experienced during an orgasm.

At the present time, research is concentrated on understanding the origin and role of the different hormones involved in the physiological processes of sexuality, and in particular during childbirth. As a result of this emphasis, we now regard the brain to be the main gland at work during the process of birth. And indeed, it is probably more important to understand where the hormones involved come from than to know the name of each of them and the ideal balance between them. However, it is nonetheless worth studying in more depth the different hormones released during the birth process, because we will recognize them as being the same ones involved in the other processes of sexuality. And this gives us an opportunity we should not miss: an opportunity to recall that sexuality is holistic. This, in turn, suggests that interfering routinely in the period around birth—as most known cultures do—probably influences the whole sexual life. According to modern science, the capacity to love is all one, singular, all of a piece, merely expressing itself in different ways.

Note

1. Electroencephalography is a technique for recording the electrical activity in different parts of the brain.

CHAPTER TWELVE

The Hormone of Love

According to modern science, there is a hormone of love. As Niles Newton has noted, wherever there is love there is oxytocin, a hormone secreted by well-defined areas of the primitive brain and released by the posterior pituitary.

For one thing, oxytocin is involved in foreplay and in male and female orgasm. It directs the orgasmic contractions of the uterus that facilitate the sucking in of the spermatic fluid and the contact between sperm and egg. Oxytocin is also released before and during suckling the baby; it initiates the milk ejection reflex. There is oxytocin in human milk, and thus the baby absorbs it when sucking. The effects of this hormone on the uterine contractions during labor are well recognized. However, the release of oxytocin peaks in the hour *after* the birth, at the time when mother and baby first make contact. Scientists have triggered maternal behavior by injecting oxytocin in precise areas of the brains of virgin animals. They have also inhibited maternal behavior by injecting into the same areas of the brain other drugs that counteract the effects of oxytocin. Interestingly, many experts believe that, through participation in the initiation of his (or her) own birth, the fetus may be training himself to secrete his own love hormone. And to all this, it should also be added that there is probably an increase in oxytocin levels during a meal — an event that is often shared with other people.

It is apparent from all these situations that oxytocin is the hormone of altruism, the forgetting of oneself. And in fact we find, significantly enough, that oxytocin depresses memory.

Of course, a hormone is always secreted in a certain context. It is never a single element, but always one part of a balanced complex. When offering the breast to her baby, a woman is not in the same hormonal equilibrium as she was when giving birth or at the moment of first contact with the newborn, or during intimate moments with her partner. The orientation of any hormonally induced altruistic state will depend on the context. The focus will vary.

Thus, the mother who is nursing her baby is in a special hormonal balance. She is under the influence of a hormone necessary for the secretion of milk: prolactin. This hormone does not only act on the breast; it is the basis for nest building in animals. It is also the hormone that triggers aggressively defensive behavior in lactating females. Studies of breastfeeding mothers and of the symptoms suffered by men and women with prolactin-secreting tumors have increased our knowledge of the behavioral effects of this hormone on humans. One such effect is the reduction of libido or sexual interest. In addition, prolactin tends to engender subordinate and submissive states of mind as well as a certain anxiety. These behavioral effects are easily explained in terms of the survival of the species. When a woman is breastfeeding, all the effects of the hormone of love are directed toward the baby. The baby becomes the object of love. The mother's subordinate state increases her adaptability to the needs of the baby. Her anxiety increases her vigilance in caring for the baby and helps prevent her from dropping into a state of deep sleep.

Given that the characteristics of a culture are shaped by the population's average hormonal balance, we should ask ourselves what is unique to our Western culture. One notable characteristic is that we have few children. Another is that the period of breastfeeding is brief, being complete in a matter of months. In most other societies, breastfeeding continues for years. In other words, high levels of prolactin are released for a very short period in the lives of Western women. In other cultures, this hormone influences the greater part of the life of an adult woman. We might conclude, therefore, that the scarcity of prolactin is unique to our society. And it is difficult to imagine that this factor would not be expressed in our collective behavior. Thus, we might have here a key to understanding ourselves better.

Let us speculate, then, on the cultural characteristics of a society where prolactin is in short supply. Certainly, in such a society, the satisfaction of the needs of the baby will not be much of a priority. And in a society where the hormone that promotes the nesting instinct is almost absent, it is to be expected that the need for privacy on the part of the woman in labor or, later, in welcoming her baby will not be recognized. An abundance of specifically erotic stimuli is to be anticipated, given that the hormone of love (oxytocin) tends to lead in only one direction when it is without the harmonizing influence of prolactin. A lack of respect for the laws of nature would be predictable. We could also expect a cavalier attitude toward natural phenomena and a tendency to "play with fire." In such a society, there is nothing to counterbalance the purely masculine brain. We must not forget that it is the dominant male who has the lowest levels of prolactin in a society of primates.

This simple line of inquiry directs us to another. What would characterize a society where prolactin is abundant? One can imagine that the attitude toward life would be very different from ours. The needs of babies and children would be respected and even given priority. Erotic stimuli would be less ubiquitous. There would probably be a great respect for the laws of nature and for destiny.

In fact, there is an existing model for such a society. It can be found among high-caste Hindus. Inside the monogamous families of this culture, children are breastfed for between three and five years. The men are traditionally priests, or *brahmin*, who spend most of their time in deep meditation. This saturates them with high levels of endorphins, and these aid the release of prolactin. It is noteworthy that these priests have an unusual physical appearance, with big breasts. Certainly, even these few facts are enough to convince us that the attitude toward life in such a society is very different from ours.

I first formulated these concerns at a conference that had brought together hundreds of breastfeeding mothers in the same room. It was as if we were in another world, with other priorities.

In considering what is cultural, we must always remember that we are taking a broader rather than an individual view. We are concerned with collective tendencies, but this does not mean that there are not individual behavioral differences. And indeed, certain individuals will exhibit behavior that does not match their physiological state. The shaping of behavior is specific to human cultures. However, we should not lose sight of the fact that cultures are made up of interactions among human beings — that is to say, separate living creatures.

These separate individuals represent the many adaptive systems used by Homo sapiens, who is a social animal. That is why our reference to the effects of certain hormones on behavior provides an opportunity to demonstrate how fragile and even artificial are the frontiers between what is biological and what is cultural.

This vision of our civilization from the perspective of the biological sciences will need to be deepened as the dawn of an ecological humanity becomes a priority — on the day when humanity stops dominating the biosphere to the point of its destruction. This is a difficult priority to develop in a society where prolactin is scarce. How can we break the vicious circle?

CHAPTER THIRTEEN

Breastfeeding and Monogamy

The circumstances are, in great measure, new. We have hardly any landmarks from the wisdom of our ancestors to guide us.

—Edmund Burke

"My baby is sick whenever I lose weight." Only a woman who has breastfed for a long time can make this observation. And only a woman who has breastfed in the context of the nuclear family of the twentieth century.

The duration of breastfeeding is a factor that, up to now, has never been taken into account when describing a particular civilization.

People have a vague feeling, for reasons they don't try to analyze, that the continuance of breastfeeding is a scandalous subject best ignored. To open up the subject would be to shake the very foundations of our society.

Any question related to the duration of breastfeeding is provocative. What is the physiological ideal for the duration of breastfeeding? For any other mammal, the answer is simple—almost as simple as for the duration of pregnancy. For example, after spending 230 days in the womb, the baby chimpanzee is fed by its mother for two years; and a bottle-nosed dolphin is breastfed for sixteen months. For human beings, the answer is much more imprecise. However, it is necessary to have some knowledge of the physiological ideal. What is physiological should be considered the reference point. To stray from this reference point is to incur the wrath of Nemesis, the goddess who punishes humans who dare to imitate the gods.

In an effort to rediscover the physiological ideal, then, we can compare human beings with other mammals and take into account the duration of our life in the womb, our degree of maturity at birth, our lifespan, the special nutritional needs of our big brain, and so forth. Such an approach will still not be precise, but it suggests that breastfeeding among humans was originally maintained for a matter of years, rather than a few months. We could also program some research into a computer, and compare individuals who have been breastfed for several months, several years, or not at all. The chosen criteria should evaluate states of health, school results, and behavior generally. No doubt, there will be an increasing number of such studies in the future. Another approach to tackling this quest might be to compare different societies and try to establish correlations. I imagine that some such correlations would be considered scandalous at first sight. Actually, however, correlations are just plain facts. And conclusions can only be scandalous when they go beyond what we know from the facts.

Let's examine the first group of such correlations we might cite. In all polygamous societies, breastfeeding is prolonged for several years. And polygamy is by far the most common marital arrangement the world over. In the 558 societies considered as representative, G. P. Murdoch found that polygamy was the norm in 76 percent. Correlating these observations leads us to two questions. First, to what extent does the polygamous society make prolonged breast-feeding easier? Second, do the long and close ties between mother and baby during prolonged breastfeeding favor the ability to share a spouse? In other words, does a short-term relationship between mother and baby exacerbate the tendency toward possessive love in the adult, making polygamy unacceptable?

The second group of correlations we might cite would specifically concern Western countries having similar standards of living, and being in geographical proximity in Northern Europe. In Sweden, where 60 percent of babies are still breastfed at six months, the rate of marital separation appears to be about 50 percent. Most of these cases occur in the first year following a birth. According to the 1986 statistics, there were 19,518 divorces and 37,017 marriages during the year. These divorces involved 21,127 children under the age of eighteen. One-fifth of the divorces, or 4,290 marriages, had lasted less than four years. In Holland, where the number of babies still breastfed at six months is extremely small, the number of separations is 25 percent. In the United Kingdom, where the rate of breastfeeding falls between these two examples, the rate of separation is also halfway between the rates for Sweden and Holland. These evaluations are approximate. There are huge differences between the rates of official and nonofficial marriages. Great Britain is one of the European countries with a high rate of official marriages; therefore, the official rate of divorce is misleading.

My attention would not have been drawn to these correlations if I had not been frequently approached in confidence by couples having difficulties during the period of prolonged breastfeeding. More often than not, trouble began with the husband's anxiety over the reduced sexual appetite of his wife. The man tends to interpret this sexual disinterest as disinterest in him. He needs to be reassured. Some men insist that their partner see a sexual therapist.

But the sex therapist does not always establish the relationship between the wife's reduced libido and her breastfeeding.

Of course, we must remember that this happens in a cultural environment where it is considered normal to have sex during pregnancy and to return to sexual activity soon after birth. When a woman leaves the maternity unit, or at the postnatal checkup, she is asked which method of contraception she prefers. This simple question is suggestive of the pressures the couple will be feeling. When a woman is breastfeeding for a long time, sometimes her behavior can be influenced by the dominant societal model. Some women claim that during the breastfeeding period their sexual relationship is more satisfying than usual. Or they might feel that their sexual appetite has not changed, but they avoid skin contact below the waist, or they need artificial vaginal lubricants, or their libido cannot easily be expressed because of pain from the episiotomy scar or because they are tired. In a culture where the only model is the nuclear monogamous family, prolonged breastfeeding can lead to some strange and uncharted situations. Some breastfeeding mothers, for example, claim that their interest in sex has returned but their husband's has not. They are anxious about being treated only as mothers, but also stress that their husband is a very good father. My interpretation of this is that in some rare cases the man's physiological state is less influenced by the cultural pattern than the woman's is. These men behave more like primates. Among other apes, the males are not sexually attracted by females who are not in a certain physiological condition. Evidently, some men can also lose their interest in sex when they become totally preoccupied with the care of young children, especially when they have participated in the birth. But, generally speaking, it is the weakened sexual appetite of lactating mothers that is underestimated or ignored in books and at conferences. And because it is not well known or understood, the reduced libido is a source of anxiety and conflict. It would often be easy to prevent or assuage this problem by giving appropriate advice and explaining that it is transitory. However, the tongues are beginning to wag; I read recently in a magazine about a woman who had "no sex drive left since the birth of her child," and who "felt strangely asexual."

Let's draw these facts together in our minds: polygamy and prolonged breastfeeding; the comparison of divorce rates in different countries; the suppressing effect of prolactin on the libido; confidential revelations by couples in difficulty during breastfeeding. Are we not obliged to pose another provocative question? Is monogamy compatible *at a cultural level* with prolonged breastfeeding?

When we talk about monogamy, we are talking about marriage. We enter a specifically human domain. In most mammalian societies — particularly those of the primates — the females have great sexual freedom. The males compete and even fight to impregnate as many females as possible. The most vigorous and dominant males, as a result, transmit the greatest number of genes. Thus, natural selection is assured. To zoologists, mammals that form monogamous relationships — such as wolves, beavers, or the small antelopes called dik-dik — are almost curiosities.

The ability to coordinate collective action such as hunting or warfare is a characteristic of the human species. This is only possible if there is a reduction in the aggression between males of the same group. Therefore the social control of sexuality. Therefore the distribution of women as mates. Therefore, at a certain stage of human evolution, marriage.

The most common form of marriage is the polygamous one. It is impossible to compile an exhaustive list of all the polygamous societies. It would be very long. It is also impossible to describe all the varieties of polygamous marriage. They are innumerable. It will be more useful to emphasize quickly some common points. In all polygamous societies, it seems, babies sleep with their mothers and breastfeed for several years — often three, or five, or even more. Sexual relations are usually forbidden for a great part of the long breastfeeding period. Indeed, there is often a separation of the sexes that begins during the pregnancy. The mother does not rejoin her husband until the baby has reached a certain age, which varies among cultures. The reunion is often celebrated.

Monogamy is another form of the social control of sexuality. It is the most common form of marriage in the industrialized world and has prevailed in Europe for about twenty centuries. Contrary to popular belief, it is not originally a Christian but a Greek–Roman phenomenon. It just so happened that the first Christians, as a general rule, adopted the form of marriage that prevailed during their time. In fact, the Bible does not contain any specific condemnation of polygamy. The cultural change occurred between the Old Testament and the New. Many examples of respectable polygamous patriarchies — for example, Abraham, Jacob, David, Solomon — can be found in the Old Testament. Similar examples cannot be found in the New Testament; the issue is not addressed at all, apart from some allusions made by Paul, particularly in his epistles to the Corinthians.

Through the centuries, in any case, Christian theologians have advocated monogamy, and the Council of Trent issued an indictment against polygamy in 1563. The majority of Christian churches refused polygamists access to the sacraments.

However, there have always been attempts to rehabilitate polygamy amongst Christians. A proclamation on polygamy was made in Münster in 1534 when the city fell under the control of Anabaptists and became a center of rigid morality where adultery and fornication were punishable by death. The Anabaptists regarded fornication as including sexual relations with one's pregnant wife. Later, in the seventeenth century, an eloquent defense of polygamy was made by Johan Leyser, a pastor and teacher who eventually sacrificed everything for his fixed idea. This scholar applied his enormous erudition exclusively to the cause of polygamy. At the same time, the famous English poet John Milton, after having campaigned in favor of divorce, became an advocate of plural marriage in an essay on his interpretation of the Christian doctrine, published posthumously in the nineteenth century. Its publication was probably instrumental in establishing the Mormon model of polygamy, and this sect provides the only example we have of a society that reestablished polygamy.

Mormon polygamy — as well as their beliefs in general — has its roots in the visions and revelations of the American prophet Joseph Smith. The revelation on polygamy officially dates from 1843; and polygamous marriage survived Smith's assassination, the abandonment of the city of Nauvoo in Illinois, and the creation of Salt Lake City in Utah. After the proclamation of extremely severe laws by the American authorities, and a number of prosecutions, a declaration by the Mormon ecclesiastics officially signaled the abandonment of polygamy in 1890. But some fundamentalists have persevered. I met a few of them in Missoula, in the state of Montana.

In Africa, where polygamy is very deeply ingrained, even some Catholic theologians understood that it is an ethnocentric error to make monogamy a prerequisite for membership in the church. It is certainly ethnocentric to impose an institution on the Africans that is more European than Christian, and that has no precise reference in the Holy Scriptures. Nevertheless, most of the Christian churches have refused the sacraments to polygamists, with the exception of some small independent churches such as a Rhodesian sect that seceded from the Seventh-Day Adventists in order to "help polygamists to enter the Kingdom of Heaven."

Those who promote this or that form of marriage — be it polygamous or monogamous — never seem to take into account the period of breastfeeding among humans. So, according to its advocates, the advantage of polygamy is its adaptability in matching the number of men to the number of women. For purely statistical reasons, it was proposed that bigamy be legalized in the Soviet Union at a time when there were 170 bachelors for every 100 spinsters. And it is because of the usual statistical distribution of men and women that polygyny (where one husband has several wives) is more frequent than polyandry (where one wife has several husbands). The polyandric societies that do exist, such as among the Toda in India, are characterized by an excess of men.

Other proponents emphasize that polygamy tends to prevent prostitution and delinquency, and to reduce the number of divorces, illegitimate children, and infanticides.

Still others focus on the side effects of monogamy they consider to be negative. So, according to Friedrich Engels, the first historical appearance of class opposition coincides with the development of the antagonism between men and women in monogamous marriages. Some feminists of the 1970s also reconsidered the institution of monogamous marriage. Barbara Leon, for example, pointed out that "smashing monogamy" was nothing new for men: "What is new, however, is its elevation to the level of an ideology."

As for those who theorize in support of monogamy, they claim that it is the only form of marriage that makes the full development of authentic marital love possible. They focus on the ties that bind the couple. Let us add that, at the present stage of medical knowledge, strict monogamy is the best possible protection against cancer of the cervix and sexually transmitted diseases.

The point of view of the breastfed baby is never given priority in all this theorizing, however. Family structures are not studied by reference to the basic needs of the human infant. If you take our mammalian nature as a starting point, if you wonder what sort of family structure would prevent enormous deviations from the physiological limits occurring during the period of breastfeeding, you have to establish unusual correlations. You have to acknowledge that all the polygamous societies permit the mother to sleep with her baby and prolong the breastfeeding for several years according to the demands of the child. You have to acknowledge that in the framework of the main monotheistic religions, with a masculine image of God, the only collection of sacred writings that gives any special importance to breastfeeding is the Koran. And the Koran permits a Muslim man to take up to four wives; it also allows his widowed, divorced, and repudiated wives to marry again. For Muslims, the first person to whom one owes veneration is one's mother, just after God and His prophet, but before one's father.

If you compare breastfeeding patterns in different family structures, you cannot help but become aware of the difficulties, and even obstacles, that seem inherent to the monogamous family and that appeared even before the evolution of the current nuclear type of family.

In Greek society there were slaves called *titthai* whose role was to breastfeed the children of their masters for six months. Women of high society were afraid of jeopardizing their health and their silhouette, and also of neglecting their "duties." In the Old Testament, during the period of transition toward monogamy, Jeremiah referred to the aversion to breastfeeding. He was talking to those who wanted to be fashionable, and who therefore refused to breastfeed, when he commented, "Even the sea monsters offer their breast to their offspring."

Yet it was still for the same reasons that women had recourse to wet nurses in Western Europe up to the nineteenth century. City women who were rich enough used to send their babies to wet nurses living in the country. These wet nurses belonged to a low socioeconomic class, and some of them were also prostitutes. Sometimes a mother would abandon her own baby or even suffocate it to devote herself to this profitable occupation. There was a time when an important chapter in every midwifery textbook dealt with how to select a good wet nurse. Let us comment that both the wet nurses and the prostitutes in monogamous societies can be thought of as mercenaries who supply substitutes for love, either maternal or marital.

The titthai, the wet nurse, and also the nursing slave in some American states were all different expressions of one same attitude that was leading to the bottle. The art of preparing a bottle became one of the most important sections in books written about childcare. Bottlefeeding hit its peak in the middle of the twentieth century, with the massive appearance on the market of industrialized powdered milks and, in particular, the so-called humanized milks.

Today, breastfeeding is coming back into favor. It is officially encouraged by doctors and public health organizations. What is unique to our own time, however, is that a majority of mothers now begins breastfeeding, but most of them do not continue for more than three to six months. Public health authorities have tried to understand why the rate of breastfeeding falls off so quickly. Some people refer to the pressures on working women. But the same phenomenon has been observed in women who do not work. Women are given plenty of advice about this postpartum era in their lives, but nobody dares to suggest that sharing their bed with the baby is the key to overcoming many difficulties they may have encountered. Nobody dares to imagine that the obstacles to prolonged breastfeeding might be inherent in the monogamous, nuclear family. To breastfeed a baby for several years, a modern woman needs to apply enormous personal resources in her effort to withstand the many social pressures that tell her to wean the child — particularly pressures from inside her own family.

Government policy making does not recognize the existence of children who are breastfed for several years. For example, in the industrialized countries, this small minority is

not taken into account in the standardized programs of im-
munization. Statistics evaluating the mortality rates during
epidemics of infectious diseases such as whooping cough
and measles do not consider how long each child may have
been breastfed.

Mothers who want to breastfeed for several years not only
have to face many difficulties thrown in their way by our society, but also have to take new kinds of precautions to avoid
impairing the baby's health — precautions that are unfamiliar and difficult to understand. Which brings us back to the
baby who gets sick whenever his or her mother loses weight.

This is an opportunity for us to elaborate on a topic that
may very well soon become a major preoccupation. Everyone who is concerned about infant feeding should focus
their attention on this phenomenon, which is quite particular to the industrialized societies.

The importance of fatty acids in human nutrition is becoming better understood. Some of these fatty acids are
called "essential" because the body cannot make them by itself. They have to be supplied via the diet. Almost all the
fatty acids found in nature share a distinctive and thus characteristic molecular shape. Chemists describe them as belonging to the "cis" series. There are a few — but very
few — exceptions to this, such as some fatty acids that are
transformed in the stomach of ruminants by local microor-
ganisms, in which case the molecule takes another shape
called "trans."

Quite suddenly, in the industrialized world, more and
more trans fatty acids have been introduced artificially into
the diet, particularly in the processing of oils and the making of margarines. Recent estimates indicate that some
Western consumers may be receiving between 7 and 10 percent of their total energy intake in the form of trans fatty
acids. But these particular fatty acids should be considered
false friends. On the one hand, they are found in foods that
are popular and even tasty; but on the other hand, they

compete with their useful counterparts and so they block some important metabolic pathways. In fact, they can be thought of as poisonous. And recently a huge amount of these trans fatty acids have been found in the breast milk of modern women. A recent study showed six times more trans fatty acids in the milk of German mothers than in the milk of African mothers taken as a control group. The rate is still higher in the United States — 1.6 times higher. This is worrisome insofar as the "good" fatty acids play an important role in the development of the baby's brain and in the composition of cell membranes. They are also the precursors of those important regulators called prostaglandins.

The dangerous fatty acids consumed by the modern baby come, of course, from the mother's diet, but not only from what the breastfeeding mother is eating. As a matter of fact, there are many such molecules in the mother's fatty deposits; and each time she loses weight, the baby consumes some more trans fatty acids. In addition, certain contaminants incorporated into modern food, such as herbicides and pesticides, are stored primarily in fatty tissues. Their release into the milk is associated with the release of the dangerous fatty acids.

These very recent data should not be taken as a reason to discourage breastfeeding. On the contrary. Along with this new information comes knowledge about the irreplaceable role of the so-called long-chain polyunsaturated fatty acids, which cannot be found in artificial milk and the importance of which has, until quite recently, been underestimated.

For practical purposes, we must conclude that pregnant women and breastfeeding mothers should learn the importance of avoiding the dangerous fatty acids. They should avoid processed oils, margarines, pastries, french fries, fast foods, and so on. There is so much at stake in this particular nutritional danger that it might perhaps be wise to advise some young mothers who cannot control their diet that they should take certain supplements, such as fish oils, that contain long-chain polyunsaturated fatty acids. Another conclusion we must draw is that losing weight when breast-feeding is not an innocuous undertaking. This brings us back to the difficulties and the contradictions that are special to the monogamous nuclear family.

However, these considerations should not be regarded as a thesis advocating any one particular family structure. We cannot be inspired by an old model at the dawn of an age when demographic growth and ecological considerations are becoming increasingly incompatible. Our objective is to stimulate a measure of reflection at this time when breast-feeding is taking a new direction. Modern science can demonstrate with authority the degree to which human milk is inimitable. We can even study different aspects of the process of attachment between mother and baby. Nowadays public health as a discipline tends to enlarge the viewpoint of medicine. It goes far beyond the treatment of diseases.

We are also at a phase of our history in which family structures are evolving rapidly and in an insidious manner. Officially we are a monogamous society, but in fact we are a society where there are two kinds of polygamy. The first of these is the so-called serial monogamy, when the man and the woman have successive spouses. This practice rightly belongs within the framework of polygamy. Knowing the rate of divorce in many Western countries, and that most divorced people remarry, one can conclude that this form of polygamy is widespread. Evidently the tendency is the same with cohabitation, which is becoming more and more common.

Then there is clandestine or semiclandestine polygamy. When Annette Lawson surveyed marriages in the American and British middle classes over a ten-year period, she was led to the conclusion that four men and four women out of five have or have had at least one second sexual partner. For women, the average time for the plunge was 4.5 years after marriage; for men, 5.2 years.

We have to be aware of these figures to be conscious of the huge changes in which we are participating. The time has come to admit that breastfeeding and family structures are two topics that cannot be studied separately. And they are issues we cannot evade any longer for fear of being thought scandalous. They necessitate the raising of new questions. What kind of family is the most appropriate to meet the basic needs of the baby of the human mammal? To what extent is the nuclear family — as a model — maintained by childbirth (and by death) in hospitals? Our ambition here has not been to find answers to such complex questions, but simply to raise the issues as straightforwardly as possible.

CHAPTER FOURTEEN

Lullaby Time

The visions presented in this book may seem outrageous at this time when the trend is toward the "humanization" of birth, as if this in itself were the priority.

To give birth to her baby, the mother needs privacy. She needs to feel unobserved. The newborn baby needs the skin of the mother, the smell of the mother, her breast. These are all needs that we hold in common with the other mammals, but that humans have learned to neglect, to ignore or even deny.

Human societies have lessons to learn from their near and distant cousins among related species.

So don't worry about humanization. On the day when human societies return to their role as protectors of the mother and baby instead of meddling in their relationship, then humanization will naturally follow. The mother will again use her hands and arms to rock the baby, and the melodies and rhythmic sounds that flow from within her will lead to a rediscovery of the specifically human lullaby.

Selected Bibliography

Introduction

Figge, D. C. "Tyranny of Technology." *American Journal of Obstetrics and Gynecology* 162, no. 6 (1990): 1365–69.

Golding, J., M. Paterson, and L. J. Kinhen. "Factors Associated with Childhood Cancer in a National Cohort Study." *British Journal of Cancer* 97 (1990): 304–8.

Jacobson, B., et al. "Obstetric Pain Medication and Eventual Adult Amphetamine Addiction in Offspring." *Acta Obstetrica Gynecologia Scandinavica* 67 (1988): 677–82.

Kellog, C. K. "Effects of Perinatal Benzodiazepines on Development of the Central Nervous System." Paper presented at the Fourth International Congress of Pre- and Perinatal Psychology. August 1989. University of Massachusetts–Amherst.

Odent, M. "Planned Home Birth in Industrialized Countries." WHO report, Copenhagen, 1991.

Chapter 2

List of the articles that suggest the electronic age in birthing is drawing to a close:

Brown, V. A., et al. "The Value of Antenatal Cardiotocography in the Management of High-risk Pregnancy: A Randomized Controlled Trial." *British Journal of Obstetrics and Gynecology* 89 (1982): 716–22.

Flynn, A. M., et al. "A Randomized Controlled Trial of Non-stress Antepartum Cardiotocography." *British Journal of Obstetrics and Gynecology* 89 (1982): 427–33.

Haverkamp, A. D., et al. "A Controlled Trial of the Differential Effects of Intrapartum Monitoring." *American Journal of Obstetrics and Gynecology* 126 (1976): 470–76.

Haverkamp, A. D., et al. "The Evaluation of Continuous Fetal Heart Rate Monitoring in High Risk Pregnancy." *American Journal of Obstetrics and Gynecology* 125 (1976): 310–20.

Kelso, I. M., et al. "An Assessment of Continuous Fetal Heart Rate Monitoring in Labor." *American Journal of Obstetrics and Gynecology* 131 (1978): 526–32.

Kidd, L. C., et al. "Non-stress Antenatal Cardiotocography — A Prospective Randomized Clinical Trial." *British Journal of Obstetrics and Gynecology* 92 (1985): 1156–59.

Leveno, K. J., et al. "A Prospective Comparison of Selective and Universal Electronic Fetal Monitoring in 34995 Pregnancies." *New England Journal of Medicine* 315 (1986): 615–19.

Lumley, J., C. Wood, et al. "A Randomized Trial of Weekly Cardiocartocography in High-risk Obstetric Patients." *British Journal of Obstetrics and Gynecology* 90 (1983): 1018–26.

MacDonald, D., I. Chalmers, et al. "The Dublin Randomized Controlled Trial of Intrapartum Fetal Heart Rate Monitoring." *American Journal of Obstetrics and Gynecology* 152 (1985): 524–39.

Prentice, A., and T. Lind. "Fetal Heart Rate Monitoring during Labour — Too Frequent Intervention, Too Little Benefit." *Lancet*, no. 2 (1987): 1375–77.

Renou, P., A. Chang, I. Anderson, and C. Wood. "Controlled Trial of Fetal Intensive Care." *American Journal of Obstetrics and Gynecology* 126 (1976): 470–76.

Sky, K., et al. "Effects of Electronic Fetal Heart Rate Monitoring, as Compared with Periodic Auscultation, on the Neurological Development of Premature Infants." *New England Journal of Medicine* (March 1, 1990): 588–93.

Wood, C. "A Comparison of Two Controlled Trials Concerning the Efficacy of Fetal Intensive Care." *Journal of Perinatal Medicine* 6 (1978): 149–53.

Wood, C., et al. "A Controlled Trial of Fetal Heart Rate Monitoring in Low-risk Obstetric Population." *American Journal of Obstetrics and Gynecology* 141 (1981): 527–34.

Other references:

Newton, N., D. Foshee, and M. Newton. "Experimental Inhibition of Labor through Environmental Disturbance." *Obstetrics and Gynecology* 27 (1966): 371–77.

Newton, N., D. Foshee, and M. Newton. "Parturient Mice: Effect of Environment on Labor." *Science* 151 (1966): 1560–61.

Chapter 3

Odent, M. *Birth Reborn*. New York: Pantheon, 1984.

Chapter 4

Schiefenhovel, W. and G. Schiefenhovel. Geburt eines Mädchens einer Primipara — Eifo (West New Guinea — Zentrales Hochland). Film E 2681, Institut Zur den Wissenschaftlichen Film, Göttingen, 1976.

Schiefenhovel, W., and G. Schiefenhovel. Vorgänge bei der Gebert eines Mädchens und Änderung der infantizid Absicht — Eifo (West New Guinea). Film E 2680, Institut Zur den Wissenschaftlichen Film, Göttingen, 1976.

Chapter 5

Embry, M. "Observations sur un accouchement terminé dans le bain." *Annales de la société de médecine pratique* 5 (1805): 13.

J-C, B. *Voyage au Canada fait depuis l'an 1751 à 1761*. Paris: Aubier-Montaigne.

Lederman, R., D. McCann, B. Work, and M. Huber. "Endogenous Plasma Epinephrine and Norepinephrine in Last-trimester Pregnancy and Labor." *American Journal of Obstetrics and Gynecology* 129 (1977): 5–8.

Newton, N. "The Fetus Ejection Reflex Revisited." *Birth* 14 (1987): 106–8.

Newton, N., and M. Newton. "Relation of the Let-down Reflex to the Ability to Breastfeed." *Pediatrics* 5 (1950): 726–33.

Odent, M. "Birth under Water." *Lancet,* no. 2 (1983): 1476–77.

Odent, M. "The Fetus Ejection Reflex." *Birth* 14 (1987): 104–5.

Odent, M. "The Role of Fear during Labour." In *Proceedings of the Ninth International Congress of Psychosomatic Obstetrics and Gynecology.* Amsterdam: Parthenon, 1989.

Odent, M. "Fear of Death during Labour." *Journal of Reproductive and Infant Psychology* 9 (1991): 43–47.

Pose, S. V., L. Cibils, and F. Zuspan. "Effect of Epinephrine Infusion on Uterine Contractility and Cardiovascular System." *American Journal of Obstetrics and Gynecology* 84 (1962): 297–306.

Dick-Read, G. *Childbirth without Fear.* London: William Heinemann, 1943.

Woodbury, R. A., et al. "The Relationship between Abdominal, Uterine and Arterial Pressures during Labor." *American Journal of Physiology* 121 (1938): 640.

Chapter 6

Van Doren, M. *Collected and New Poems, 1924–1963.* New York: Hill and Wang, 1963.

Chapter 7

Aucher, M. L. "Les maternités chantantes." Volume 5 of *L'Aube des sens — Cahiers du nouveau-né.* Paris: Stock, 1981.

Hardy, A. "Was Man More Aquatic in the Past?" *New Scientist* 7 (April 1960): 642–45.

Kramer, R. *Maria Montessori: A Biography.* Oxford: Basil Blackwell, 1976.

Lorenz, K. *Studies in Animal and Human Behavior.* Cambridge: Cambridge University Press, 1971.

Lorenz, K. Vergleichende Verhaltensforschung: Grundlagen der Ethologie. Wien: Springer-Verlag, 1978.

Mellers, W. *Bach and the Dance of God.* London: Faber and Faber, 1980.

Odent, M. *Genèse de l'homme écologique.* Paris: Epi, 1979.

Odent, M. "What Is Health? Towards an Ontogenic Definition." *International Journal of Prenatal and Perinatal Studies* (1989): 47–49.

Odent, M. *Water and Sexuality.* Hammondsworth, UK: Penguin, 1990.

Chapter 8

Baumslag, N. *Breastfeeding: Cultural Practices and Variations.* Volume 7 of *Advances in International Maternal and Child Health.* Oxford, UK: Clarendon, 1987.

Bullough, C. H. W., et al. "Early Sucking and Post Partum Haemorrhage: Controlled Trial in Deliveries by Traditional Birth Attendants." *Lancet,* no. 2 (1989): 522–25.

Cadogan, W. "Essay on Nursing and Management of Children from Birth to Three Years of Age." Letter to One of the Governors of the Foundling Hospital, Published by Order of the General Committee of the Said Hospital, London, 1773. Reprinted in Volume 7 of *Advances in International Maternal and Child Health,* ed. D. B. Jeliffe and E. F. Jeliffe. London: Clarendon, 1987.

Gartner, L. M. "Breastfeeding in Korea." *Breastfeeding Abstracts,* La Leche League, vol. 7, no. 2 (1987).

Gibson, R. A. "Fatty Acid Composition of Human Colostrum and Mature Breast Milk." *American Journal of Clinical Nutrition* 34 (1981): 252–57.

Hamilton, A. *Nature and Nurture.* Canberra: Australian Institute of Aboriginal Studies, 1981.

Jordan, B. *Birth in Four Cultures.* Montreal: Eden Press, 1980.

Mead, M., and N. Newton. "Cultural Patterning in Perinatal Behavior." In *Childbearing: Its Social and Psychological Aspects,* ed. S. Richardson et al. Baltimore: Williams and Williams, 1967.

Odent, M. "Newborn Weight Loss." *Mothering* (January 1989): 72–74.

Shaw, E., and J. Darling. *Female Strategies.* New York: Simon and Schuster, 1986.

Tildes, V. *Breasts, Bottles and Babies — A History of Infant Feeding.* Edinburgh, UK: Edinburgh University Press, 1986.

Chapter 9

Bullough, C. H. W., et al. "Early Sucking and Post Partum Haemorrhage: Controlled Trial in Deliveries by Traditional Birth Attendants." *Lancet,* no. 2 (1989): 522–25.

Kloosterman, G. J. "The Dutch Experience of Domiciliary Confinements." Pp. 115–25 in *Pregnancy Care for the 1980s,* L. G. Zander and G. Chamberlain, eds. London: Royal Society of Medicine and Macmillan, 1984.

Newton, N. "Some Aspects of Primitive Childbirth." *Journal of the American Medical Association* 188 (1964): 261–64.

Odent, M. "In Praise of the Traditional Birth Attendant." *Lancet,* no. 2 (1989): 861–62.

Tew, M. *Safer Childbirth.* New York: Chapman and Hall, 1990.

Treffers, P. E., and R. Laan. "Regional Perinatal Mortality and Regional Hospitalization at Delivery in the Netherlands." *British Journal of Obstetrics and Gynecology* 93 (1986): 690–93.

Van Altan, D., M. Eskes, and P. E. Treffers. "Midwifery in the Netherlands: The Wormerveer Study." *British Journal of Obstetrics and Gynecology* 96 (1989): 656–62.

Chapter 11

For the African Yorube midwifery poem displayed at the beginning of the chapter:

Priya, J. V. *Birth Traditions and Modern Pregnancy Care.* Dorset, UK: Element Books, forthcoming 1992.

For other references:

Kennel, J., M. Klaus, S. McGrath, S. Robertson, and C. Hinkley. "Continuous Emotional Support during Labor in a U.S.

Hospital." *Journal of the American Medical Association* 265, no. 17 (May 1, 1991): 2197–2201.

Cohen, Nancy. *Open Season*. New York: Bergin & Garvey, 1992.

Nilsen, S. T. "Boys Born by Forceps and Vacuum Extraction Examined at 18 Years of Age." *Acta Obstetrica Gynecologia Scandinavica* 63, no. 6 (1984): 549–54.

Roemer, F., et al. "Retrospective Study of Fetal Effects of Prolonged Labor before Cesarean Delivery." *Obstetrics and Gynecology* 77, no. 5 (1991): 653–58.

Seidman, D., et al. "Long Term Effects of Vacuum and Forceps Deliveries." *Lancet* 337 (1991): 1583–85.

Sosa, R., J. Kennel, M. Klaus, S. Robertson, and J. Urrutia. "The Effect of a Supportive Companion on Perinatal Problems, Length of Labor, and Mother-Infant Interaction." *New England Journal of Medicine* 303 (1980): 597–600.

Chapter 12

Arletti, R., et al. "Oxytocin Improves Copulatory Behavior in Rats." *Hormones and Behavior* 19 (1985): 14–20.

Egli, G. E., and M. Newton. "Transport of Carbon Particles in the Human Female Reproductive Tract." *Fertility and Sterility* 12 (1961): 151–55.

De Wied, D. "Memory Effects of Oxytocin and Related Peptides." In *Proceedings of the Ninth International Congress of Psychosomatic Obstetrics and Gynecology*. Amsterdam: Parthenon, 1989.

Newton, N. "The Role of the Oxytocin Reflexes in Breastfeeding." In *Clinical Psychoneuro-endocrinology in Reproduction: Proceedings of the Second Symposia*. Orlando, FL: Academic Press, 1978.

Newton, N., and C. Modahl. "New Frontiers of Oxytocin Research." In *Proceedings of the Ninth International Congress of Psychosomatic Obstetrics and Gynecology*. Amsterdam: Parthenon, 1989.

Takeda, S., Y. Kuwabara, and M. Mizuno. "Concentrations and Origin of Oxytocin in Breastmilk." *Endocrinology Japan* 33 (1986): 821–26.

Uvnas-Moberg, K. "Hormone Release in Relation to Physiological and Psychological Changes in Pregnant and Breastfeeding

Women." In *Proceedings of the Ninth International Congress of Psychosomatic Obstetrics and Gynecology.* Amsterdam: Parthenon, 1989.

Verbalis, J. C., et al. "Oxytocin Secretion in Response to Cholecystokinin and Food." *Science* 232 (1986): 1417–19.

Chapter 13

Cairncross, J. *After Polygamy Was Made a Sin: The Social History of Christian Polygamy.* London: Routledge and Kegan Paul, 1974.

Chappell, J. E., et al. "Trans Fatty Acids in Human Milk: Influence of Maternal Diet and Weight Loss." *American Journal of Clinical Nutrition* 42 (1985): 49–56.

Engels, F. *The Origin of the Family, Private Property and the State.* London: Lawrence and Wishart, 1982.

Finley, D. A., et al. "Breastmilk Composition: Fat Content and Fatty Acid Composition in Vegetarians and Non-vegetarians." *American Journal of Clinical Nutrition* 41 (1985): 787–800.

Hillman, E. *Polygamy Reconsidered: African Plural Marriage and the Christian Churches.* Maryknoll, NY: Orbis, 1975.

Koletzko, B., et al. "Fatty Acid Composition of Mature Milk in Germany." *American Journal of Clinical Nutrition* 47 (1988): 954–55.

Lawson, A. *An Analysis of Love and Betrayal.* London: Basil Blackwell, 1989.

Leonard, J., A. Leonard, and D. Leonard. *The Mormon Experience: A History of the Latter-Day Saints.* New York: Random House, 1980, p. 200.

Mayer, J. F. "Etre chretien . . . et polygame?" *Rebis* 9 (1985).

Murdoch, G. P. "Marriage." In *Encyclopaedia Universalis,* volume 13, 1972, p. 234.

Odent, M. *Genèse de l'homme ecologique.* Paris: Epi, 1979.

Van Wert, W. F. "Sex after Children." *Mothering* (Summer 1991): 115–17.

Index

ABOUT THE AUTHOR

MICHEL ODENT is Director of Research for the Primal Health Research Center in London and former Director of the Maternity Unit in the French State Hospital in Pithiviers, France.